Essentials of
Cardiovascular
Physiology

Essentials of
Cardio
Phys

University of Minnesota Press □ Minneapolis

Harvey V. Sparks, Jr., M.D.

Professor and Chairman
Department of Physiology
Michigan State University

and

Thom W. Rooke, M.D.

Fellow, Mayo Graduate School of Medicine
Mayo Clinic/Mayo Foundation
Stanley J. Sarnoff Fellow
for Research in Cardiovascular Science

vascular ology

Original illustrations by
ROBERT R. LORENZ

Editorial preparation of manuscript by
JULIANNE O. ROOKE

Published by the University of
Minnesota Press, 2037 University
Avenue Southeast, Minneapolis
MN 55414.
Published simultaneously in
Canada by Fitzhenry & Whiteside
Limited, Markham.
Printed in the United States of
America.

**Library of Congress
Cataloging-in-Publication Data**
Sparks, Harvey V., 1938-
    Essentials of cardiovascular
physiology.

    Includes bibliographies and
index.
    1. Cardiovascular system.
I. Rooke, Thom W.
II. Title. [DNLM: 1. Cardiovascular
System—physiology.
WG 102 S736e]
QP102.S684 1987 612.1 86-7011
ISBN 0-8166-1472-5
ISBN 0-8166-1473-3 (pbk.)

Publication of this book was
assisted by a grant from the
McKnight Foundation to the
University of Minnesota Press's
program in the health sciences.

To Barbara and Julie

Contents

Figures

Tables

Preface

Medical educators and students must cope with an exponential increase in knowledge, but no additional time to learn. Our goal was to write an introductory text that can be read and understood in the two- to three-week period most curricula provide for cardiovascular physiology. An understanding of this subject requires knowledge of facts and concepts ranging from membrane channels and contractile proteins to the cardiovascular correlates of behavior. Our task was to select those facts and concepts that are essential to a solid initial comprehension of the subject. When we had to choose between presenting a clear concept or acquainting the reader with our current state of confusion, we almost always chose the former. We believe that once the student has an overall grasp of the subject he or she will be ready to accept and understand a more complex view that includes the many exceptions to the rule we have laid out and, equally important, the clinical applications of the material.

We have made the most significant points both in the text and in the figures, and so the figures should be useful for rapid review. The references were chosen to lead the student to expanded treatments of the subjects covered in each chapter, and from there to the original literature. We have also pointed the way to the history of cardiovascular sciences, with the hope that some students will have the time and curiosity to find out who is responsible for all that is known.

H.V.S./T.W.R.

Acknowledgments

We are indebted to those who assisted in the preparation of this book, particularly Mrs. Agnes Osborn, whose dedication and perseverence helped make this project possible. We also greatly appreciate the assistance of our colleagues from Michigan State University who read and had constructive comments on portions of the text, Joseph R. Hume, Ph.D., Houria I. Hassouna, M.D., Ph.D., and Lana Kaiser, M.D.

Essentials of
Cardiovascular
Physiology

Chapter 1

Once Around
the Circulation

Almost every physiological process involves the maintenance of the milieu interieur (internal environment), or *homeostasis*. This internal environment is determined by the composition of fluid surrounding the cells of various organs and tissues. Optimal cellular function requires that the characteristics of this fluid remain within certain limits despite wide variations in the external environment. Consequently, variables such as the partial pressure of gases, the concentration of many organic and inorganic substances, and temperature must be regulated with precision. In higher organisms, different regulatory functions are performed by anatomically separate organs and tissues; for example, the lungs regulate gas concentrations, the splanchnic organs control the uptake and metabolism of a variety of organic and inorganic substances, and the skin is especially important in temperature regulation. Because the cells of every organ and tissue require access to all of these regulating capacities, a system of transport between each site of regulation and the cellular environment must be present. The circulation of the blood provides this system and enables homeostasis to be achieved.

SYSTEMIC AND PULMONARY CIRCULATION

The human cardiovascular system consists of (1) two pumps in series, the left and right hearts; and (2) two corresponding vascular tracts, the systemic and pulmonary circulations (fig. 1-1). As blood returns from the lungs, it is pumped by the left heart into the aorta at a mean hydrostatic pressure of approximately 93 mmHg above atmospheric (intravascular pressure is defined as the hydrostatic pressure of blood above or below atmospheric pressure at heart

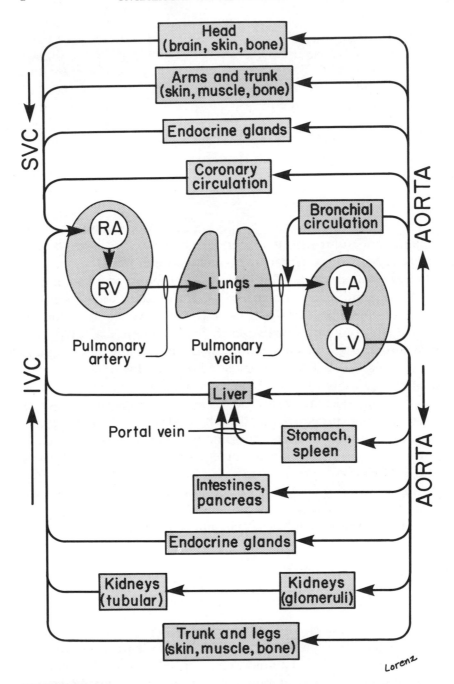

FIGURE 1-1.
Schematic outline of the cardiovascular system. RA = right atrium, RV = right ventricle, LA = left atrium, LV = left ventricle, IVC = inferior vena cava, SVC = superior vena cava.

level, but in general usage the reference to atmospheric pressure is dropped and the difference is referred to simply as the blood pressure). The pressure forces blood from the aorta into large arteries, small arteries, arterioles, and finally the vessels with the smallest diameter, the *capillaries*. As it returns to the heart, blood flows from the capillaries into the venules, small veins, large veins, superior and inferior vena cavae, and finally to the right atrium. This general scheme applies for each of the multiple parallel circuits (e.g., brain, kidney, gut) that compose the systemic circulation. The right atrial blood pressure is close to 0 mmHg, so the approximate pressure difference driving blood through the systemic circulation is 93 mmHg (aortic minus right atrial pressure). Because of the parallel distribution system, capillaries in most tissues receive blood with a composition identical to that of blood in the aorta.[1]

Blood flows from the right atrium into the right ventricle, where it is pumped into the pulmonary arteries. Here the blood pressure averages 13 mmHg. As in the systemic circulation, blood flows through the pulmonary arteries, arterioles, capillaries, venules, and veins. From the pulmonary veins it enters the left atrium, where the average blood pressure is 5 mmHg. The approximate pressure difference driving blood through the lungs is therefore 8 mmHg (pulmonary arterial minus left atrial pressure). This small difference reflects the very low resistance to blood flow offered by the vasculature of the lungs.

TRANSPORT

The cardiovascular system employs two types of transport: *diffusion* and *bulk flow*. Diffusion is accomplished by the random movement of individual molecules and is an effective transport mechanism over short distances. It occurs primarily at the level of the capillaries, where the distances between the blood and the surrounding tissue are short. The net transport of molecules by diffusion can occur within hundredths of a second or less when the

---

[1]There are three notable exceptions to this. (1) Blood draining the gut and splenic capillaries enters a second set of capillaries in the liver; this is referred to as the *hepatic portal circulation*. (2) In the kidney, blood first traverses the glomerular capillaries and then enters the peritubular capillaries. (3) Blood from the hypothalamic capillaries passes directly to the capillaries of the anterior pituitary; this is the *hypothalamic portal circulation*. In each instance as the blood passes the first set of capillaries it undergoes exchange with the surrounding extracellular fluid. This exchange alters the composition of the blood with respect to the partial pressure of gases, nutrient content, etc., and as a consequence the second set of capillaries receives blood that can differ substantially from that in the aorta.

distances involved are no more than a few micrometers. On the other hand, minutes or hours would be needed for diffusion to occur over millimeters or centimeters.

The circulation of the blood is an example of transport by bulk flow. Bulk flow requires a pressure difference, with the fluid (in this case blood) flowing from an area of high to low pressure. This is an efficient means of transport over long distances, such as those between the legs and the lungs. In summary, the cardiovascular system depends upon the energy provided by a concentration gradient to move material over short distances (diffusion) and the energy provided by a pressure gradient to move materials over long distances (bulk flow).

Table 1-1 describes the physical characteristics of mesenteric

Table 1-1.
Geometrics, Flow Velocities, and Pressures in the Mesenteric Circulation (Approximate)

Structure	Diameter, mm	Number	Total Cross Section, cm²	Length, cm	Mean Linear Flow Velocity, cm/sec	Mean Pressures, mmHg Prox.	Distal	Δ
Aorta	10.0	1	3	50.0	35.0	94	92	2
Terminal arteries	0.6	3,600	10	1.0	7.0	89	83	6
Arterioles	0.02	80,000,000	250	0.2	0.3	83	35	48
Capillaries	0.005	2,400,000,000	1200	0.1	0.05	35	15	20
Venules	0.03	160,000,000	1140	0.2	0.06	15	8	7
Terminal veins	1.5	3,600	60	10.0	1.0	8	5	3
Inf. vena cava	2.5	1	4	50.0	23.0	3	2	1

blood vessels. Other vascular beds have similar characteristics. The aorta has the largest diameter of any artery, and the subsequent branches become progressively smaller until the capillaries are reached. Although the capillaries are the smallest blood vessels, the total cross sectional area of the lumens of all capillaries greatly exceeds the cross sectional area of the lumen of the aorta (1200 cm² vs. 3.12 cm²). In a steady state, the total blood flow must be equal at any point along the circulation. Because of this, total flow is the same through the aorta and the capillaries; however, the combined cross sectional area of the capillaries is much greater, so the velocity of flow in the capillaries is much lower. This enables blood to move slowly through the capillaries and provides the maximum opportunity for diffusional exchange of substances between blood and extracellular fluid. In contrast, blood moves quickly in the aorta, where bulk flow transport, as opposed to exchange, is important.

BLOOD

Blood consists of red blood cells, white blood cells, and platelets suspended in plasma. The cells make up approximately 45% of the total blood volume (roughly 5.8 L in a 70-kg individual).

Red blood cells (*erythrocytes*) are biconcave discs approximately 7.5μm in diameter and 2μm thick. There are approximately 3×10^{13} circulating erythrocytes in the average person. The cells are red because they contain the oxygen-carrying protein, *hemoglobin*, which is red when combined with oxygen. The hemoglobin in the red blood cells raises the oxygen-carrying capacity of blood from approximately 3.0 mL to 198 mL of oxygen per liter of blood. Without hemoglobin, the erythrocytes would be unable to transport sufficient oxygen to sustain life.

White blood cells (*leukocytes*) are present in smaller numbers than erythrocytes. There are normally 4,000-11,000 white blood cells per microliter of blood as compared with 5 million erythrocytes in the same volume. White blood cells can be divided into three types. *Granulocytes* comprise approximately 50% to 70% of the leukocyte population. The most common form of granulocytes (*neutrophils*) search out, ingest, and kill organisms that invade the body. Neutrophils are capable of leaving the blood and entering tissue by squeezing through the gaps in the walls of the capillaries and venules. The other two forms of granulocytes (*eosinophils* and *basophils*) are thought to be involved in allergic (hypersensitivity) reactions. *Monocytes*, another type of leukocyte, can enter the tissues from the blood and eventually transform into tissue macrophages; these ingest bacteria or other foreign bodies. The remaining type of leukocyte is the *lymphocyte*, an important component of the body's immune system.

Platelets are small fragments of cytoplasm pinched off from the giant cells in the bone marrow. Platelets contain several substances including prostaglandins, phospholipids, vasoconstricting agents, platelet-derived growth factors, and two platelet-specific proteins: platelet factor 4 and β-thromboglobulin. The platelet is important in the control of hemostasis and may also play a role in a variety of pathophysiological conditions, such as the development of atherosclerosis obliterans.

Plasma, the fluid in which the blood cells are suspended, is a complex solution containing numerous ions, inorganic molecules, amino acids, fats, and proteins. The plasma proteins include albumin, various types of globulins, and fibrinogen; these make up about 7% of the plasma volume. Some plasma proteins are hormones and antibodies, while others serve as carriers of small compounds such as lipids, certain hormones, or drugs.

HEMOSTASIS

When a small blood vessel is severed, loss of blood is terminated by a series of events that proceed from release of tissue thromboplastin to platelet adhesion and vasoconstriction (fig. 1-2). Disruption of the endothelial cells lining the vessel exposes underlying collagen, to which platelets will adhere. Platelet adhesion is followed by activation and release by platelets of serotonin, adenosine diphosphate (ADP), and thromboxane A_2. ADP and thromboxane A_2 cause other platelets to aggregate, forming a plug that fills the opened vessel.

Constriction of the injured blood vessel results from contraction of the smooth muscle in its wall in response to agents released from platelets. These agents include serotonin and thromboxane A_2. *Prostacyclin* is released by endothelial cells and inhibits platelet aggregation.

The formation of *fibrin* from its soluble precursor *(fibrinogen)* is initiated by the release of tissue *thromboplastin* (a protein-lipid complex) from injured cells. Fibrinogen circulates in plasma and is hydrolyzed by *thrombin*, a serine protease, to form fibrin. The cascade of reactions responsible for the generation of thrombin from prothrombin will not be covered in detail. Active factor X (in the presence of Ca^{2+}, platelet phospholipids, and factor V) converts prothrombin to thrombin. Thrombin cleaves the fibrinogen molecule so that fibrin monomers are formed. These polymerize to form fibrin, and the intertwining strands of fibrin polymers are then converted to a dense meshwork by crosslinking reactions catalyzed by factor XIII.

The powerful clotting mechanism is held in check by anticoagulant proteins and by the *fibrinolytic system*. The major inhibitor of thrombin is *antithrombin III*, which functions as a heparin cofactor in plasma. *Heparin* lines the inner surface of blood vessels and catalyzes the inhibition of thrombin by antithrombin III. *Fibrinolysin (plasmin)* digests fibrin and induces clot lysis.

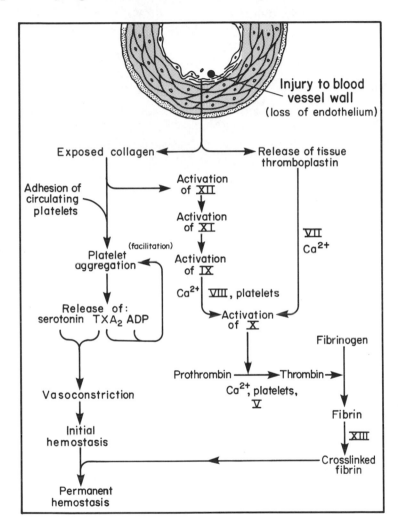

FIGURE 1-2.
Effect of injury on blood vessels. Injury to the blood vessel wall results in disruption of endothelium and exposure of underlying collagen. Collagen plus thromboplastin from the blood vessel wall cause a cascade of reactions leading to fibrin formation. Collagen also stimulates platelet aggregation, and platelets release vasoconstrictors such as serotonin and thromboxane A_2. Vasoconstriction, platelet aggregation, and fibrin deposition lead to the permanent hemostatic plug that terminates bleeding.

Suggested Readings

Burton AC: Why have a circulation? In *Physiology and Biophysics of the Circulation*. 2d ed. Chicago, Yearbook Medical Publishers, 1972, pp 3-14

Cournand A: Air and blood. In *Circulation of the Blood: Men and Ideas*. Edited by AP Fishman and DW Richards. Bethesda, American Physiological Society, 1982, pp 3-70

Hamilton WF, Richards DW: The output of the heart. In *Circulation of the Blood: Men and Ideas.* Edited by AP Fishman and DW Richards. Bethesda, American Physiological Society, 1982, pp 71-126

Ganong WF: Circulating body fluids. In *Review of Medical Physiology*. 12th ed. Los Altos, CA, Lange Medical Publications,1985, pp 421-441

Ratnoff OD: Blood. In *Physiology*. Edited by RM Berne and MN Levy. St. Louis, The C. V. Mosby Company, 1983, pp 407-438

Chapter 2

Electrical Activity of the Heart

The heart will beat in the absence of any nervous connections because the electrical (pacemaker) activity that generates the heartbeat resides within the heart itself. After initiation, the electrical activity spreads in a coordinated manner (electrical conduction) through a network of specialized cells and tissues distributed throughout the heart. The electrical activity reaches every cardiac cell rapidly and with the correct timing, thus enabling the contraction of individual cells to occur in a coordinated fashion.

The electrical pacemaker and conduction properties of cardiac cells depend upon the ionic gradients that exist across their semipermeable membranes. This chapter describes how ionic gradients and changes in membrane permeability result in the electrical activity of individual cells, and how this electrical activity is propagated throughout the heart.

IONIC BASIS FOR ELECTRICAL ACTIVITY

MEMBRANE POTENTIAL OF CARDIAC CELLS

The inside of a cardiac cell at rest has a negative potential (voltage) when compared with the outside. This difference in electrical potential across the cell membrane is the *membrane potential*. In ventricular muscle cells, the resting membrane potential (labeled 4, meaning Phase 4, in fig. 2-1A) is stable at approximately -90 mV. When the cell is appropriately stimulated, a transient change in the membrane potential occurs. First, there is a rapid increase (phase 0) from -90 mV to $+20$ mV. This is followed by a slight decline (phase 1) to a plateau (phase 2) when the membrane potential nears zero, and finally a rapid return (phase 3) of potential to the resting value (phase 4). The sequence of phases 0 to 4 is called the *action potential.*

In contrast, changes in the membrane potential of the cells of the sinoatrial (SA) node (fig. 2-1B) are characterized by a progressive depolarization during phase 4 (or diastole) called the *pacemaker potential*. When the membrane potential reaches a characteristic

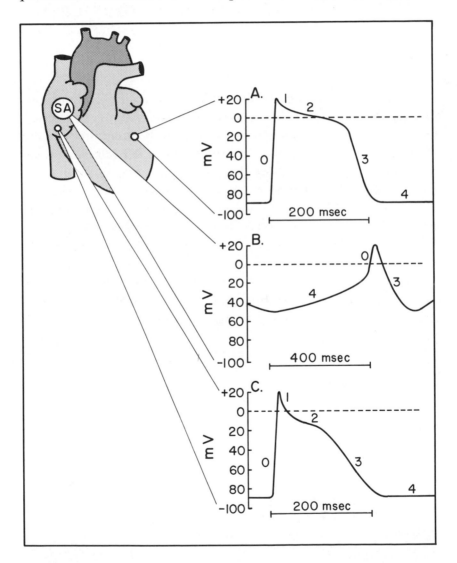

FIGURE 2-1.
Cardiac action potentials. Action potentials (mV) are recorded from (A) ventricular, (B) sinoatrial, and (C) atrial cells. Note difference in time scale of B.

voltage (the threshold potential), there is a sudden and rapid depolarization (phase 0) to approximately + 20 mV. The membrane subsequently repolarizes (phase 3) and the pacemaker potential
resumes (phase 4). Other myocardial cells combine various characteristics of the electrical activity of these two cell types. Atrial cells,
for example (fig. 2-1C), have a steady diastolic resting membrane
potential (phase 4) but lack a definite plateau (phase 2). Cells of the
atrioventricular (AV) node are the only myocardial cells other than
those of the SA node that normally have pacemaker potentials.

MOLECULAR BASIS OF CATION MOVEMENTS ACROSS CARDIAC CELL MEMBRANES

The backbones of cardiac cell membranes are phospholipids arranged in a bilayer with their hydrophobic regions directed toward
the interior of the membrane (fig. 2-2). The phospholipid bilayer is
not permeable to charged hydrophilic molecules the size of K^+,
Na^+, or Ca^{2+}. These cations move across the membrane by means of
various membrane proteins that serve as carriers or channels for
particular cations.

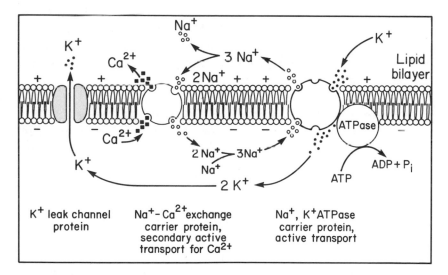

FIGURE 2-2.
Transport of K^+, Ca^{2+}, and Na^+ by membrane proteins. These cations cannot
cross the lipid bilayer in the absence of carrier and/or channel proteins. Movements of cations via channels obey the laws of simple diffusion. In general,
movement via carrier proteins obeys laws similar to those that govern enzyme reactions.

Carrier proteins bind the cations and move them across the membrane by changes in the configuration of the protein. The change in configuration requires chemical energy that can be supplied, either by the gradient(s) of one or more of the cations, or by ATP. When an electrical or concentration gradient supplies the energy, the transport of an ion down its electrochemical gradient is referred to as *facilitated diffusion*. A good example of this is the movement of Na^+ into cardiac cells via a carrier protein that exchanges Na^+ for Ca^{2+} (fig. 2-2). A second form of carrier protein-mediated transport is *active transport.* Here the energy to transport an ion against its electrochemical gradients comes from the splitting of ATP. An example of this type of protein is *Na^+,K^+ ATPase*. This protein extrudes 3 Na^+ from the cell for every 2 K^+ transported into the cell. The energy required for the conformational change of the carrier protein is derived from ATP (fig. 2-2).

Sometimes an ion is transported against its electrochemical gradient by a carrier protein that obtains the chemical energy required for conformational changes from the concentration gradient of a second ion. This is called *secondary active transport*. An example of this is the extrusion of Ca^{2+} from cardiac cells (by the carrier protein mentioned above, which also transports Na^+ into the cell [fig. 2-2]). The extrusion of Ca^{2+} against its electrochemical gradient is accomplished by conformational changes in the carrier protein, which are energized by the transport of Na^+ down its electrochemical gradient.

Another class of membrane proteins that transport cations across the cell membranes is *channel proteins*. These proteins provide hydrophilic pathways through the lipid bilayer and allow cations to move by simple diffusion down their concentration gradient. Some of these channels are opened or closed by changes in membrane potential *(voltage-gated channels)*, or by changes in the concentration of neurotransmitters, hormones, or drugs *(ligand-gated channels)*. An example of a voltage-gated channel is the fast Na^+ channel. This channel opens as the membrane potential rises above threshold (fig. 2-3). The resultant increase in permeability to Na^+ is responsible for the sharply rising phase 0 of the action potential. A good example of a ligand-gated channel is found in the smooth muscle of blood vessel walls. These cells have Ca^{2+} channels that open in response to norepinephrine; Ca^{2+} then enters these cells by diffusing down its electrochemical gradient.

Many of the drugs used in the treatment of cardiovascular diseases exert their effects by acting upon the various carrier and channel proteins.

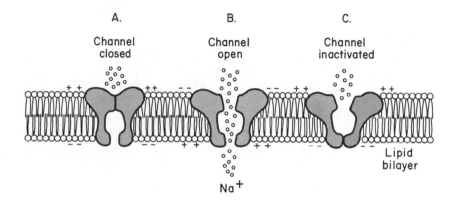

FIGURE 2-3.
Activation of Na$^+$ channels. The fast Na$^+$ channel is closed when the membrane is normally polarized (A). It opens when the membrane is depolarized to threshold (B). It is inactivated for a time after opening (C) and cannot be reopened until it returns to its resting closed state (A). The inactivated state is responsible for the refractory period.

REFRACTORY PERIOD

During most of the action potential, cells are refractory to further excitation; that is, additional stimuli will not initiate action potentials. This occurs because the fast Na$^+$ channels become inactive for a period of time after having been opened (fig. 2-3). Figure 2-4 reveals that the membrane potential must return almost halfway to the normal resting potential before the cardiac cell is responsive to stimuli of any magnitude (*effective* or *absolute refractory period*). From the end of the absolute refractory period until repolarization is completed, the cell can be excited only by strong, artificial stimulation (*relative refractory period*). The long duration of the refractory period ensures that cardiac muscle cannot develop prolonged, tonic contractions (tetanus) as can occur in skeletal muscle. Although this means that the heart cannot develop as much force as skeletal muscle, it eliminates the possibility that a sustained contraction might occur and prevent the cyclic contractions required to pump blood.

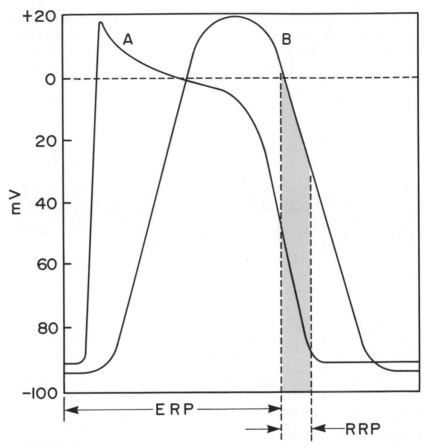

FIGURE 2-4.
Tension development in ventricular muscle. A relationship exists between the action potential (A) and the isometric tension curve (B) of isolated ventricular muscle. Note that muscle has begun to relax when the effective refractory period (ERP) is over and is even more relaxed after the relative refractory period (RRP).

IONIC BASIS FOR THE CARDIAC MEMBRANE POTENTIAL

The membrane potential of myocardial cells results from transmembrane concentration gradients for Na^+, K^+, and Ca^{2+}. The gradients are maintained through the transport of these cations via the membrane protein carriers. If the energy supply of the cell is restricted by inadequate blood flow to the myocardium, active transport may be impaired. This can result in a reduction of the ionic concentration gradients and eventually disrupt the electrical activity of the heart.

Active transport keeps the K^+ concentration high, and the Na^+ and Ca^{2+} concentrations low, in the cell cytosol. These cations tend to diffuse across the membrane down their electrochemical gradients via the protein channels. The K^+ leak channels in the resting membrane are open, and the permeability to K^+ is therefore much higher than it is to Na^+ and Ca^{2+}. As K^+ diffuses from the cell, it leaves behind less permeable anions, creating a negative intracellular charge. K^+ continues to leave the cell until the force of the negative intracellular charge (which opposes further diffusion) increases enough to offset the force from the K^+ concentration gradient (which favors further diffusion). Because the entry (or exit) of any cation will likewise affect the intracellular charge, the magnitude of the intracellular potential depends upon the relative permeability of the membrane to Na^+, Ca^{2+}, and K^+. When the membrane is much more permeable to K^+ than to Na^+ or Ca^{2+} (as occurs in the resting state), the measured potential is close to the potential that would exist if the membrane were permeable only to K^+ *(potassium equilibrium potential)*. When the membrane is more permeable to Na^+ than to the other ions, the measured potential is closer to the potential that would exist if the membrane were permeable only to Na^+ *(sodium equilibrium potential)* (fig. 2-5). Specific changes in the number of open channels conducting the various ions are responsible for changes in permeability during the different phases of the action potential.

MEMBRANE CHANGES IN VENTRICULAR CELLS

Figures 2-6 and 2-7 depict the membrane changes that occur in ventricular cells. The initial upswing of the action potential (phase 0) occurs when electrical charges from an external source or adjacent area of the cell bring the membrane potential to *threshold*. Threshold is defined as the membrane potential at which the Na^+ permeability suddenly increases while the K^+ permeability decreases. These permeability changes result from the opening of fast Na^+ channels and the closing of K^+ leak channels. As the permeability to Na^+ exceeds that to K^+, the membrane potential approaches the sodium equilibrium potential (a positive value). The change in the membrane potential from rest toward the sodium equilibrium potential is called *depolarization*. As Na^+ enters the cell, the positive charges repel intracellular K^+ ions into nearby areas where depolarization has not yet occurred; K^+ is even driven into adjacent

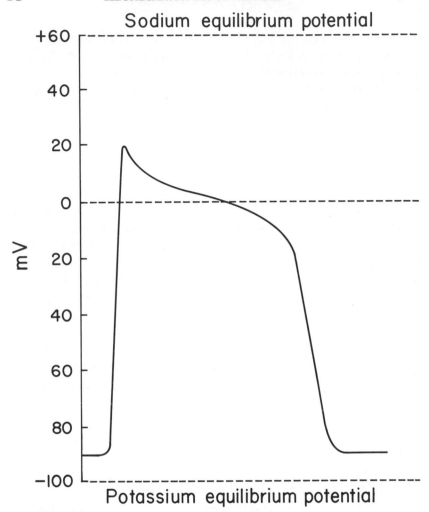

FIGURE 2-5.
Effect of ionic permeability on membrane potential. Membrane potential is determined by the relative permeability of the membrane to Na^+ and K^+. Relatively high permeability to K^+ places the membrane potential close to the potassium equilibrium potential, and relatively high permeability to Na^+ places it close to the sodium equilibrium potential.

resting cells through low-resistance areas of the intercalated disc.[1] This movement of K^+ ions depolarizes these adjacent areas until threshold is reached. The cycle of depolarization (to threshold), Na^+ entry, and subsequent displacement of positive charges into nearby areas producing depolarization explains the propagation of the action potential within (and between) cells.

[1]*Intercalated discs* are the end-to-end junctions of myocardial cells; the low resistance areas are the *gap junctions.*

The ionic basis for the remainder of the action potential is unproven, but the following events are probably important. Phase 1 may be related to a decrease in the number of open fast Na^+ channels. The plateau (phase 2) results from a combination of low membrane permeability to K^+ and an increased permeability to Na^+ and Ca^{2+}.[2] The return of the membrane potential to the resting state (phase 3) reflects the closing of Na^+ and Ca^{2+} channels and the opening of K^+ channels.

MEMBRANE CHANGES IN NODAL CELLS

When the electrical activity of a cell from the SA node is compared with that of a ventricular muscle cell, two important differences are observed: (1) the presence of a pacemaker potential and (2) the lack of a well-defined plateau. The pacemaker potential results from a steady decrease in the membrane permeability to K^+ during diastole (phase 4) caused by the closing of K^+ leak channels. Since permeability to Na^+ remains unchanged, the reduced permeability to K^+ moves the membrane potential toward the sodium equilibrium

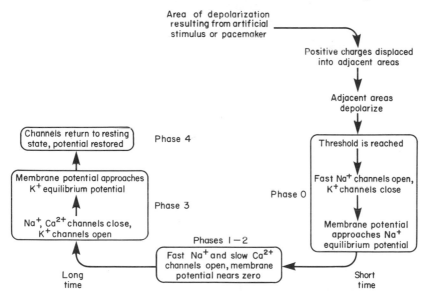

FIGURE 2-6.

Events associated with the action potential. Note that events between phases 0 and 1, and between phases 2 and 3 are time dependent, rather than a direct result of the previous step.

---

[2]Ca^{2+} entering the cell during the action potential couples excitation to contraction (see chapter 3). The calcium equilibrium potential, like that for sodium, is positive. Increased permeability to Ca^{2+} moves the membrane potential away from the potassium equilibrium potential and toward the sodium equilibrium potential.

potential; that is, it becomes less negative. An action potential is triggered when threshold is reached. The absence of a well-defined plateau is probably due to the continued presence of a relatively high permeability to K^+ throughout the action potential.

The pacemaker cells of the SA and AV nodes are under the influence of nerves from the *parasympathetic* (releasing acetylcholine) and *sympathetic* (releasing norepinephrine) *nervous systems*. Acetylcholine slows the heart rate *(bradycardia)* by reducing the

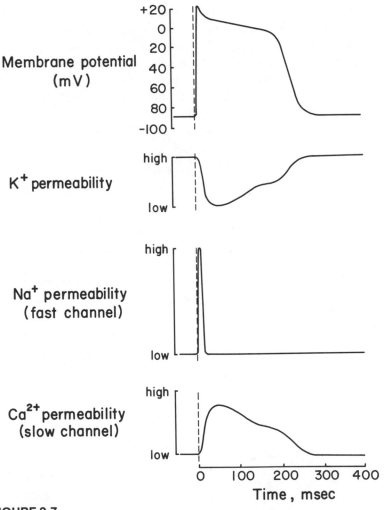

FIGURE 2-7.
Changes in cation permeabilities during a Purkinje fiber action potential. Compare with fig. 2-6.

rate of spontaneous depolarizations of the pacemaker cells (fig. 2-8), thereby increasing the time required to reach threshold and initiate an action potential. Acetylcholine exerts this effect by increasing the number of open K^+ channels, which holds the membrane potential closer to the potassium equilibrium potential. In contrast, norepinephrine causes an increase in the slope of the pacemaker potential so that threshold is reached more rapidly and the heart rate increases *(tachycardia)*. Norepinephrine increases the slope of the pacemaker potential by opening channels for Na^+ and Ca^{2+}, which results in faster movement of the membrane potential toward the sodium equilibrium potential.

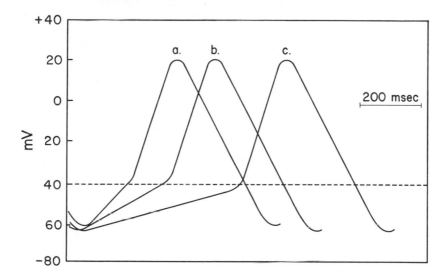

FIGURE 2-8.
Sinoatrial cell membrane potential. Normal pacemaker potential (b) is affected by norepinephrine (a) and acetylcholine (c). The dashed line indicates threshold potential.

PROPAGATION OF ELECTRICAL ACTIVITY

CONDUCTION OF THE ACTION POTENTIAL

The low-resistance gap junctions of the intercalated discs allow the entire myocardium to depolarize rapidly as the action potential is propagated from cell to cell. The heart is said to be a *functional syn-cytium* because the excitement of one cardiac cell eventually results in the excitement of all cells. During *antegrade conduction* the action potentials originating in the atria are propagated to the ventricles via the AV node. An abnormal action potential originating in the ventricles may likewise be propagated to the atria via *retro-grade conduction*. The AV node appears capable of retrograde conduction in many normal individuals; however, the extent to which this occurs under normal physiological conditions is still debated.[3]

Excitation of the heart normally begins in the SA node (fig. 2-9A)

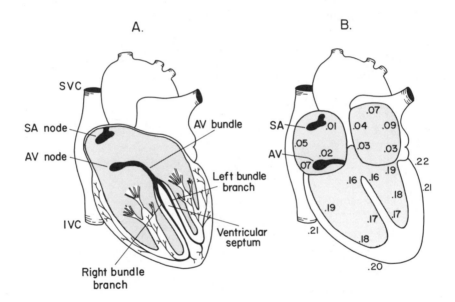

FIGURE 2-9.
Electrical conduction in the heart. (A) The specialized conducting system of the heart. (B) Timing of excitation of various areas of the heart (in fractions of a second).

because the pacemaker potential of this tissue reaches threshold before the pacemaker potential of the AV node. The intrinsic pacemaker rate of the SA node is approximately 70 beats per minute, whereas the pacemaker rate of the AV node is approximately 30 beats per minute. Many cells of the SA node reach threshold and depolarize almost simultaneously, creating a voltage difference between these cells (depolarized) and nearby resting cells

[3]In certain pathophysiological situations, retrograde conduction through or around the AV node does occur. This may give rise to a variety of *tachyarrhythmias,* the best known of which is the *Wolff-Parkinson-White* syndrome.

(polarized). The voltage difference generates the flow of cations mentioned earlier and brings the adjacent cells to threshold, initiating their action potentials. Excitation proceeds as succeeding cycles of local ion current and action potentials move in an enlarging circle over the atria from the SA node. This process is referred to as the *propagation of the action potential*. It requires 60-90 msec to excite all regions of the atria (fig. 2-9B) with excitation proceeding at a speed of approximately 1 m/sec.

A fibrous, nonconducting connective tissue ring separates the atria from the ventricles everywhere except at the AV node. Because of the nonconducting ring, the transmission of electrical activity from the atria to the ventricles occurs through the AV node. Action potentials in the atrial muscle adjacent to the AV node produce local ion currents that invade the node and trigger intranodal action potentials. The propagation of the action potential by local current flow continues within the AV node, but at a much slower velocity (0.05-0.1 m/sec). The slow velocity of conduction is explained by the small size of the nodal cells and the fact that less current is produced by the depolarization of a small nodal cell than a large myocardial cell.[4] Propagation of the action potential through the AV node takes approximately 120 msec. Excitation then proceeds through the AV bundle (bundle of His), the bundle branches, and the Purkinje system. The AV node is the weak link in the excitation of the heart. Inflammation, hypoxia, parasympathetic neural activity, and certain drugs (e.g., digitalis, beta blockers, and calcium entry blockers) can cause failure of the AV node to conduct some or all of the atrial depolarizations to the ventricles. This same tendency for slow conduction is of benefit in pathological situations where atrial depolarizations are too frequent (atrial fibrillation or flutter). In these conditions, not all of the electrical impulses that reach the AV node are conducted to the ventricles, and the ventricular rate tends to stay below the level where diastolic filling is impaired (see chapter 3).

The Purkinje system is composed of specialized myocardial cells with large diameters and high conduction velocities (up to 2 m/sec) that rapidly propagate the electrical activity throughout the subendocardium of both ventricles. Depolarization then proceeds from

---

[4]When large cells depolarize, they produce more electrical current than do small cells. The relatively greater current causes neighboring cells to depolarize more quickly, and the associated rate of propagation is rapid.

endocardium to epicardium as indicated in fig. 2-9B. Conduction velocity through ventricular muscle is 0.3 m/sec, and complete excitation of both ventricles takes approximately 75 msec.

THE ELECTROCARDIOGRAM

The *electrocardiogram* is a continuous record of cardiac electrical activity obtained by placing sensory electrodes on the surface of the body and recording the potential differences generated by the heart. An *electrocardiograph* amplifies these differences and causes a pen to deflect in proportion to them on a paper moving under the pen at 25 mm/sec. When the electrocardiograph is properly calibrated, a 1 mV voltage difference between two points on the body produces a 1 cm deflection of the pen. There are several combinations of points on the body from which the electrocardiogram is routinely recorded. The standard (bipolar) limb leads record the potential differences between the left and right arm (lead I), the left leg and right arm (lead II), and the left arm and leg (lead III) as shown in fig. 2-10. By convention, the electronics are arranged so that the pen makes an upward deflection when the first named point is positive relative to the second named point (e.g., when the left arm is positive relative to the right arm). Since the arms and legs act as conductors, the electrodes of the electrocardiogram recorder can be attached to them at any location.

To interpret the electrocardiogram, it is necessary to understand the behavior of electrical potentials in a three-dimensional conductor of electricity. Consider what happens when wires are run from the positive and negative terminals of a battery into a tub containing salt solution (fig. 2-11). Positively charged ions will flow toward the negative wire (negative pole) and negatively charged ions will simultaneously flow in the opposite direction toward the positive wire (positive pole).[5] The flow of ions (current) is greatest in the region between the two poles, but some current flows at every point; this reflects the fact that voltage differences exist everywhere in the solution.

What points encircling the dipole in fig. 2-11 have the greatest voltage difference between them? Points A and B do, because A is

---

[5]The combination of two poles that are equal in magnitude but opposite in charge, and that are located in close physical proximity to one another, is called a dipole.

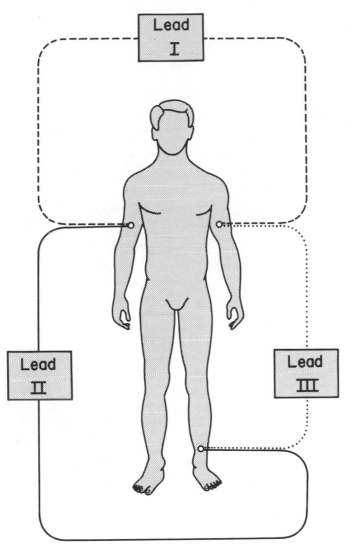

FIGURE 2-10.
Standard ECG limb leads.

closest to the positive pole and B is closest to the negative pole. Positive charges are drawn from the area around point B by the negative end of the dipole, which is relatively near. The positive end of the dipole is relatively distant and therefore has little ability to attract negative charges from point B (although it can draw negative charges from point A). As positive charges are drawn away, point B is left with a net negative charge (or negative voltage). In contrast, the

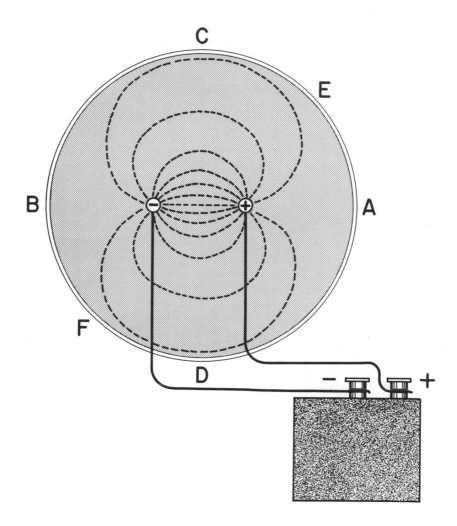

FIGURE 2-11.
Creation of a dipole in a tub of salt solution.

opposite event is happening between the positive end of the dipole
and point A, leaving A with a net positive charge (or voltage).

Points C and D have no voltage difference between them because they are equally distant from both poles and therefore are
equally influenced by positive and negative charges. Any other two
points on the circle, E and F for example, have a voltage difference
between them that is less than the voltage difference between A and
B, and greater than the voltage difference between C and D. This is

also true of other combinations of points such as A and C, B and E, and D and F. Voltage differences exist in all cases and are determined by the relative influences of the positive and negative ends of the dipole.

What would happen if the dipole were to change its orientation relative to points C and D? Figure 2-12 shows a recording of the changes that would occur as the dipole is rotated 90 degrees so that

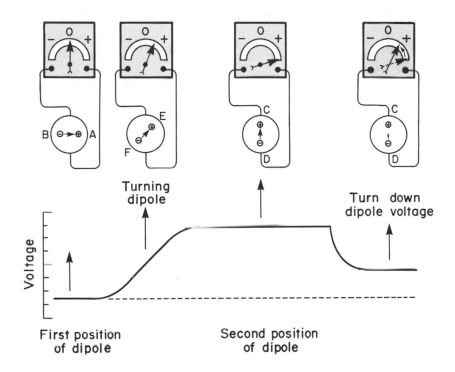

FIGURE 2-12.
Magnitude and direction of a dipole. In a salt solution, the dipole can be represented as a vector having a length and a direction that are determined by the dipole magnitude and position, respectively. When the vector is directed parallel to a line between A and B, no voltage is measured. When the vector is directed parallel to a line between C and D, the voltage is maximum. If the magnitude of the vector is decreased, the voltage decreases.

the positive end of the dipole points directly at C and the negative end at D. The voltage increases slowly as the dipole is turned and is maximal when the dipole reaches the new position. This figure also shows that the voltage between points C and D will decrease to a new steady state level as the voltage applied to the wires by the battery is decreased. These imaginary experiments illustrate two characteristics of a dipole that determine the voltage measured at distant points in a volume conductor: (1) *direction* of the dipole relative to the measuring points and (2) *magnitude* (voltage) of the dipole.

Next consider the origin of the cardiac voltage changes that are recorded as the electrocardiogram. At rest, myocardial cells have a negative charge inside and a positive charge outside the cell membrane. As the cell depolarizes, the depolarized portion becomes negative on the outside, whereas the region ahead of the depolarized portion remains positive on the outside (fig. 2-13). Once the entire cell depolarizes, no voltage differences exist between any outside areas of the cell. When the cells in a given region depolarize synchronously, as occurs during normal excitation, that portion of the heart becomes a dipole. The depolarized portion constitutes the negative side, and the yet-to-be depolarized portion the positive side of the dipole. The tub of salt solution is analogous to the rest of the body, creating a dipole in a volume conductor. With electrodes located at various points around the volume conductor (i.e., the body), the voltage resulting from the dipole generated by the electrical activity of the heart can be measured.

Consider the voltage changes produced by a two-dimensional model in which the body serves as a volume conductor, and the heart generates a continuously changing dipole (fig. 2-14). An electrocardiographic recorder is connected between points A and B. By convention, when point A is positive to point B the electrocardiogram is deflected upward, and when B is positive relative to A a downward deflection results. The solid arrows show (in two dimensions) the magnitude and direction of the actual dipoles. The lengths of the arrows are proportional to the mass of myocardium generating the dipole. The open arrows show the magnitude of the dipole component that is parallel to a line between points A and B; this component determines the voltage that will be recorded on the electrocardiogram.

Atrial excitation results from a wave of depolarization that originates in the SA node and spreads over the atria as indicated in panel 1. The dipole generated by the excitation has a magnitude proportional to the mass of the atrial muscle involved and a direction indicated by the solid arrow. The head of the arrow points toward the positive end of the dipole, where the atrial muscle is not yet depolarized. The negative end of the dipole is toward the tail of the arrow,

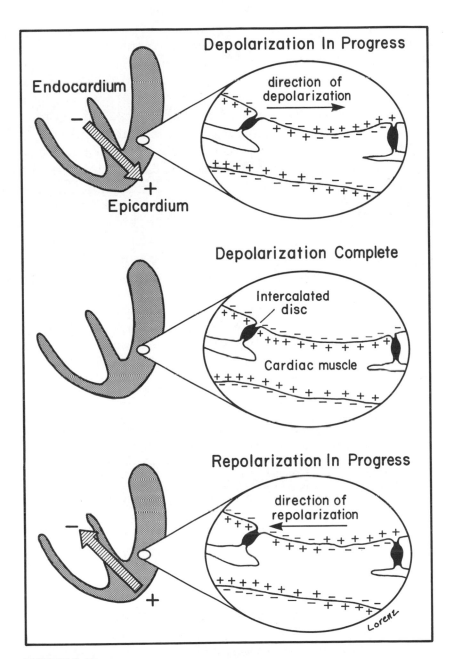

FIGURE 2-13.
  Cardiac dipoles. Partially depolarized or repolarized myocardium creates a dipole. Arrows show the direction of depolarization (or repolarization). Dipoles are present only when myocardium is undergoing depolarization or repolarization.

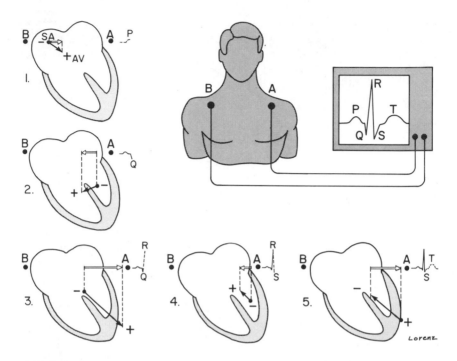

FIGURE 2-14.

Sequence of major dipoles giving rise to electrocardiographic waveforms. In each panel the solid arrow is a vector that represents the magnitude and direction of a major dipole. The magnitude is proportional to the mass of myocardium involved. The direction is determined by the orientation of polarized and depolarized regions of the myocardium. The vertical dashed lines project the vector onto the A-B coordinate; it is this component of the vector that is sensed and recorded (open arrow).

Note that in 5 the orientation of the solid arrow reflects the direction of repolarization (as opposed to depolarization, shown in figs. 2-1 through 2-4). The head of this arrow represents the yet-to-be repolarized region of the myocardium (negative), and the tail represents the region that has already repolarized (positive). By convention, the projected vector (open arrow) points so that its head is directed toward the more positive electrode (A) as opposed to the less positive electrode (B).

where depolarization has already occurred. Point A is therefore positive relative to point B, and there will be an upward deflection of the electrocardiogram as determined by the magnitude and direction of the dipole. Once the atria are completely depolarized no voltage difference exists between A and B, and the voltage recording returns to zero. The voltage change associated with atrial excitation appears on the electrocardiogram as the *P wav*e.

As conduction moves slowly through the AV node, the mass of tissue involved is too small to create a dipole with sufficient magnitude to produce a voltage difference on the electrocardiogram. The depolarization wave emerges from the AV node and travels along the atrioventricular bundle, bundle branches, and Purkinje system; these tracts extend down the interventricular septum. The direction of the resulting dipole is shown in panel 2. Point B is positive relative to point A because the left side of the septum depolarizes before the right side. The small downward deflection that this produces on the electrocardiogram is called the *Q wave.* The normal Q wave is often so small that it is not apparent.

The wave of depolarization spreads via the Purkinje system across the inside surface of the ventricles. Depolarization of the ventricular muscle proceeds from the inner muscle layer (endocardium) to the outer layer (epicardium). The muscle mass of the left ventricle is much greater than the mass of the right ventricle, and the net dipole during this phase has the direction indicated by panel 3. The deflection of the electrocardiogram is upward because point A is positive relative to point B, and it is large because of the great mass of tissue involved. This upward deflection is the *R wave.*

The voltage returns to zero as all of the ventricular muscle becomes depolarized and the dipole disappears. The last portion of the ventricle to depolarize is near the atria, and the direction of the dipole associated with this phase is shown by panel 4. Point B is positive compared with point A, and the deflection on the electrocardiogram is downward. This final deflection is the *S wave.*

The Q, R, and S waves *(QRS complex)* show the progression of ventricular muscle depolarization. Once all of the ventricular muscle is depolarized no potential differences (dipoles) exist and the electrocardiogram is said to be *isoelectric* (zero voltage). At this point all of the ventricular muscle cells are in the plateau phase (phase 2) of the action potential (fig. 2-15).

Repolarization, like depolarization, generates a dipole because the voltage of the depolarized area is different from the voltage of the repolarized areas. The dipole associated with atrial repolarization does not appear as a separate deflection on the electrocardiogram because it occurs during ventricular depolarization and is masked by the greater deflections (QRS complex) that are present at this time. Ventricular repolarization occurs well after the QRS complex and is not as orderly as ventricular depolarization. Unlike

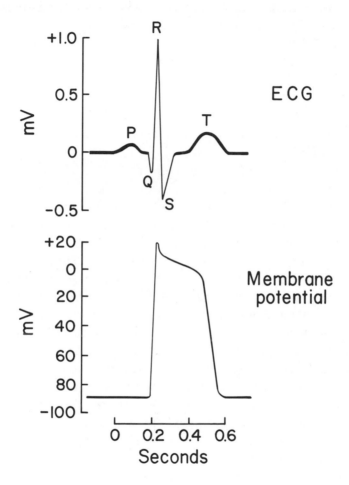

FIGURE 2-15.
Timing of ventricular potential and ECG. Note that the ST segment occurs during the plateau of the action potential.

depolarization, repolarization proceeds from the epicardial to the endocardial surface of the ventricles. One explanation for this difference is that cold blood returning from the extremities cools the endocardial surface, and this slows repolarization and prolongs the plateau of the ventricular muscle action potential. As a consequence, repolarization begins at the warmer epicardial surface and proceeds inward. Although the direction of repolarization (epicardium to endocardium) is opposite to that associated with depolarization (fig. 2-13), the polarity of the dipole is the same. This happens because the epicardium of the ventricle is positive on the outside (having repolarized first) at a time when the endocardium is still negative. As in depolarization, point A is positive with respect to point B, and an upward deflection occurs on the electrocardiogram. This deflection is the *T wave* (fig. 2-14).

Several *unipolar* leads are routinely recorded along with the standard ones. The designation "unipolar" means that most of the electrical activity is due to voltage differences on only one side of the lead. For example, the unipolar chest leads are obtained by connecting the three limb leads and recording the difference between their combined voltage and the voltage at various points on the chest (fig. 2-16).[6] The voltage changes due to the sum of the three limb electrodes are considered to be zero, and the voltage differences recorded by the unipolar leads are therefore the result of voltage changes on the surface of the chest. This permits the electrical activity generated by various parts of the heart to be examined in more detail by measuring voltages from areas of the chest wall that are nearby. By convention, an upward deflection of the pen indicates that the unipolar (exploring) electrode is positive with respect to the three combined electrodes. Unipolar chest leads are designated V_1 through V_6, and they are traditionally placed over the areas of the chest shown in fig. 2-17.

Three other routinely recorded leads are aV_R, aV_L, and aV_F ("a" stands for augmented). These give the voltages between electrodes on two of the limbs (averaged to yield a reference potential) and the third limb. For example, lead aV_F gives the potential difference between the left and right arm (interconnected) and the left foot. The exploring electrode in this case is the one attached to the left foot. The use of multiple leads ensures that the magnitude and direction of the cardiac dipole can be accurately determined no matter how it changes with time.

---

[6]The three limb leads are actually interconnected to one another and attached to a recorder through a large resistor. Electronic filtering is also done to reduce noise and give a stable baseline. Details like this will be omitted to simplify the explanations.

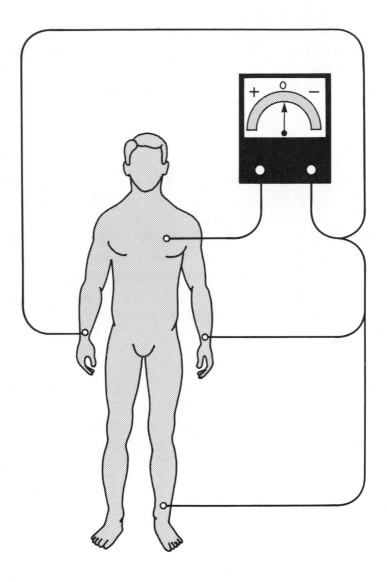

FIGURE 2-16.
Unipolar chest lead. Three limb leads are combined to give the reference voltage (zero).

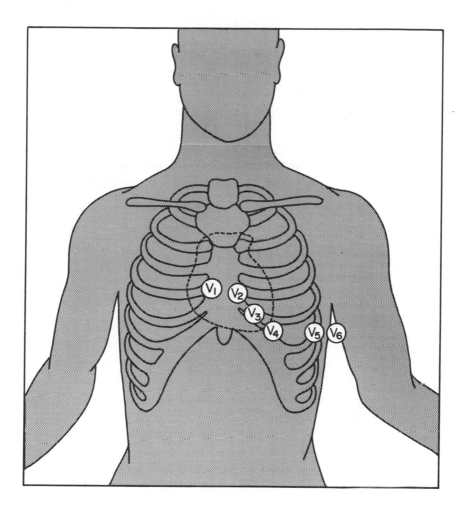

FIGURE 2-17.

Positions of the unipolar chest leads. V_1 is just to the right of the sternum in the fourth intercostal space. V_2 is just to the left of the sternum in the fourth interspace. V_4 is in the fifth interspace in the midclavicular line. V_3 is midway between V_2 and V_4. V_5 is in the fifth interspace in the anterior axillary line. V_6 is in the fifth interspace in the midaxillary line.

INTERPRETATION OF THE ELECTROCARDIOGRAM

The electrocardiogram provides information about (1) the pattern of excitation of the heart, (2) changes in the mass of electrically active myocardium, and (3) abnormal dipoles resulting from injury to the myocardium. The electrocardiogram gives no direct information about the mechanical effectiveness of the heart. (Other tests, which will be described in chapter 3, must be used to assess the efficiency of the heart as a pump.)

Examples of the first type of information are shown in fig. 2-18, where the electrocardiogram from a normal individual is compared with those from persons with variations in the normal pattern of cardiac excitation (arrhythmias). Panel A is a 12-lead electrocardiogram from an individual with *normal sinus rhythm*. The P wave (atrial excitation) is always followed by a QRS complex of uniform shape and size. The PR interval (beginning of the P wave to beginning of the QRS complex) is 0.18 sec (normal range: 0.10-0.20 sec). This indicates that the conduction velocity of the action potential from the SA node to the ventricular muscle is normal. The average time between R waves (successive heart beats) is about 0.8 sec, making the heart rate approximately 75 beats per minute.

Panel B shows the electrocardiogram of a child with *sinus arrhythmia*. Sinus arrhythmia is an increase in the heart rate with inspiration and a decrease with expiration. The presence of a P wave before each QRS complex indicates that these beats originate in the SA node. Intervals between successive beats of 0.90, 0.86, 0.80, and 0.76 seconds correspond to heart rates of 66, 70, 75, and 79 beats per minute. The duration between the beginning of the P wave and the end of the T wave is uniform, and the change in the interval between beats is primarily accounted for by the variation in time between the end of the T wave and the beginning of the P wave. Although the heart rate changes, the interval during which electrical activation of the atria and ventricles occurs does not change nearly as much as the interval between beats. Sinus arrhythmia is caused by the small cyclic changes in neural activity to the heart that accompany respiration.

Panel C shows the electrocardiogram during excessive stimulation of the parasympathetic nerves. The stimulation releases acetylcholine from nerve endings in the SA node; this suppresses the pacemaker activity, slows the heart rate, and increases the distance between P waves. The third QRS complex is not preceded by a P wave because the ventricles are excited by an impulse that originated in the AV node. This occurs because acetylcholine suppresses the activity of the SA node below that of the AV node, making the AV node the primary pacemaker (sinus arrest). When a QRS complex

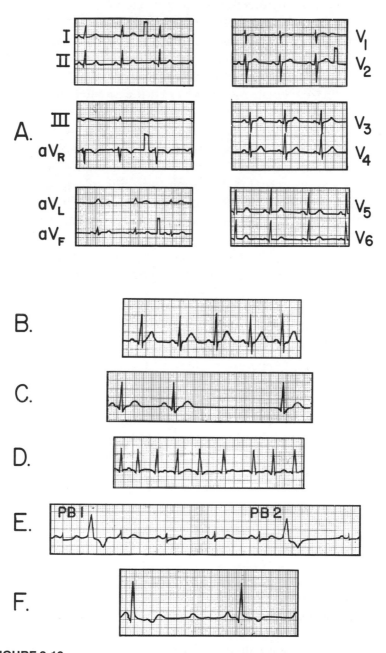

FIGURE 2-18.
Normal and abnormal electrocardiograms. (A) Normal 12-lead electrocardiogram. (B) Sinus arrhythmia. (C) Sinus arrest with vagal escape. (D) Atrial fibrillation. (E) Ventricular premature beats. (F) Complete atrioventricular block.

takes place without a preceding P wave, it reflects the fact that ventricular excitation occurs without a preceding atrial contraction. This phenomenon is *vagal escape*. The interval between the last atrial beat and the escape beat is 2.6 sec, which is equivalent to a heart rate of 23 beats per minute and consistent with the observation that the AV pacemaker activity has a firing rate between 15 and 35 beats per minute.

Panel D is an electrocardiogram from a patient with *atrial fibrillation*. In this condition atrial systole does not occur because the individual cells are electrically excited at random. As a result, there are always some excited cells among those located near the AV node, and each nodal cell will be excited as soon as its refractory period ends. The result is a ventricular rate that is rapid and irregular. Atrial fibrillation is associated with numerous disease states, such as cardiomyopathy, pericarditis, hypertension, and hyperthyroidism.

Panel E is an electrocardiogram showing *premature ventricular beats* (PB_1 and PB_2). Following a normal QRS complex, a complex of increased voltage and longer duration occurs (PB_1, PB_2). The premature beat is not preceded by a P wave, and it may be followed by a pause before the next normal P wave and QRS complex. The premature ventricular excitation is initiated by an *ectopic focus*. An ectopic focus is an area of pacemaker activity in other than the SA node. In the previous example of excessive parasympathetic stimulation (panel B), the ectopic focus was in the AV node. In this case it is probably in the Purkinje system or ventricular muscle, where an aberrant pacemaker activity reaches threshold before being depolarized by the normal wave of excitation (ectopic foci can also be in the atria). Once the ectopic focus triggers an action potential, the excitation is propagated over the ventricles and into the AV node. The abnormal pattern of excitation accounts for the greater voltage (change of dipole direction) and longer duration (inefficient conduction) of the QRS complex. Retrograde conduction often dies out in the AV node, so the atria are not excited. The normal atrial excitation (P wave) occurs, but is hidden by the abnormal QRS complex. This P wave does not result in ventricular excitation because the AV node is still refractory when the impulse arrives. As a consequence, the next "scheduled" ventricular beat is missed. The prolonged interval following a premature ventricular beat is the *compensatory pause*. In some circumstances the AV node is not refractory when the next atrial excitation occurs, and a premature ventricular excitation occurs between normal ventricular contractions. In this case the premature ventricular beat is called an *extrasystole*.

Panel F is an electrocardiogram in which both P waves and QRS complexes are present, but they appear to occur independently. This is *atrioventricular block*. The AV node fails to conduct impulses from the atria to the ventricles, and since this is the only electrical connection between these areas, the pacemaker activities of the two become entirely independent. In this particular example the atrial rate is near 75 while the ventricular rate is only 29 beats per minute. The atrial pacemaker is probably in the SA node, and the ventricular pacemaker is probably in some portion of the atrioventricular conducting system. In certain conditions the PR interval is lengthened, but all atrial excitations are eventually conducted to the ventricles. This is *first degree atrioventricular block*. If some, but not all, of the atrial excitations are conducted by the AV node, it is *second degree atrioventricular block*. If atrial excitation never reaches the ventricles, as in this example, it is *third degree (complete) atrioventricular block.*

CHANGE IN MASS

The recordings from leads I, II, and III in fig. 2-19 show the effect of right ventricular enlargement on the electrocardiogram. The increased mass of right ventricular muscle changes the direction of the major dipole during ventricular depolarization, resulting in large, inverted QRS complexes in leads I and II. This illustrates how a change in the mass of excited tissue can affect the amplitude and direction of the QRS complex.

ABNORMAL DIPOLES

If a portion of the ventricular myocardium fails to receive sufficient blood flow (injury), the supply of ATP may decrease below that required to maintain the active transport of ions across the cell membrane, and this might affect the electrocardiogram. There are normally two periods when no dipoles exist: (1) the interval between the completion of the T wave and the onset of the P wave, during which repolarization is complete (diastole); and (2) the interval between the end of the QRS complex and the onset of the T wave, during which depolarization is complete (systole). These periods are normally recorded as zero voltages on the electrocardiogram. When the supply of ATP in an area of myocardium becomes

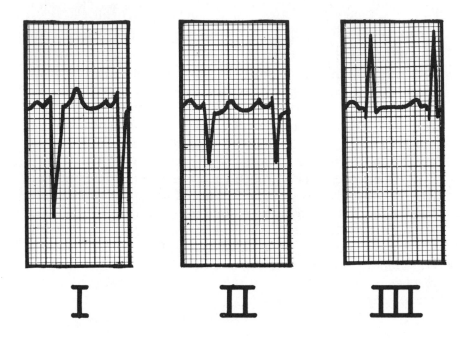

FIGURE 2-19.

ECG of patient with right ventricular hypertrophy.

limited, the ability of the cells to sustain a normal resting membrane potential is impaired, although their ability to depolarize appropriately is well maintained. As a consequence, a dipole develops at rest (TP interval) in injured hearts because of the voltage differences between normal and abnormal tissue. This dipole will cause either an upward or downward deflection on the electrocardiogram, depending upon where the injured tissue is and which leads are examined. No dipole occurs during the ST interval because depolarization is uniform and complete in both injured and normal tissue. An area of injury, for example, might therefore produce a downward deflection during the TP interval, but not during the ST interval. However, the electrocardiogram is designed so that the TP interval is recorded as zero voltage. As illustrated in fig. 2-20, this causes the ST interval to be recorded as an upward deflection. These deflections during the ST interval are of major clinical importance in the diagnosis of cardiac injury or ischemia.

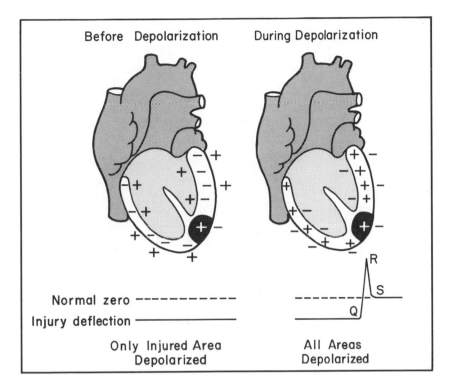

FIGURE 2-20.
Electrocardiogram changes in myocardial injury. ST segment elevation can occur with myocardial injury. The apparent zero baseline of the ECG before depolarization is below zero because of partial depolarization of the injured area. After depolarization (during the action potential plateau) all areas are depolarized and the true zero is recorded. Because zero baseline is set arbitrarily (on the ECG recorder), one cannot distinguish between a depressed diastolic baseline and an elevated ST segment. Regardless of the mechanism, this is referred to as an elevated ST segment.

Suggested Readings

Berne RM, Levy MN (eds.): *Cardiovascular Physiology*. 4th ed. St. Louis, The C. V. Mosby Company, 1981, pp 5-51

Katz AM: *Physiology of the Heart*. New York, Raven Press, 1977, pp 229-353

Katz LN, Hellerstein HK: Electrocardiography. In *Circulation of the Blood: Men and Ideas*. Edited by AP Fishman and DW Richards. Bethesda, American Physiological Society, 1982, pp 265-354

Sperelakis N: *Physiology and Pathophysiology of the Heart*. Boston, Martinus Nijhoff, 1984

Chapter 3

The Heart as a Pump

The heart is a muscular organ that pumps blood throughout the circulation. It consists of a series of four separate chambers (two atria and two ventricles) that use one-way valves to direct blood flow. The ability of the heart to pump blood depends upon the integrity of the valves and the proper contraction of the muscular walls. An understanding of the physiology of cardiac muscle is therefore a prerequisite for understanding the performance of the heart as a pump. This chapter describes (1) the basic molecular mechanisms underlying the contraction of cardiac muscle, (2) various factors that can influence these mechanisms, and (3) the performance of the intact heart.

MOLECULAR BASIS OF CARDIAC MUSCLE CONTRACTION

The heart consists of long, thin muscle fibers (actually cells) that branch and join other fibers at intercalated discs (fig. 3-1). Within each fiber are the elements responsible for contraction; these are called *myofibrils*. Each myofibril is composed of repeating structures called *sarcomeres*, which are the functional units of muscle contraction. Each sarcomere contains a large number of thick and thin filaments. The thin filaments are attached to structural proteins at each end of the sarcomere *(Z-line)*, and the thick filaments are arranged so that each of them is surrounded by six thin filaments (fig. 3-1). On a microscopic level, thick and thin filaments slide past one another as contraction occurs. The molecular mechanism responsible for the sliding of filaments will be described later, after a brief discussion of the chemical nature of the thick and thin filaments.

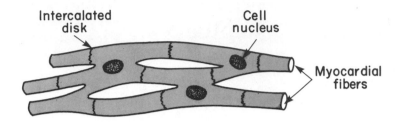

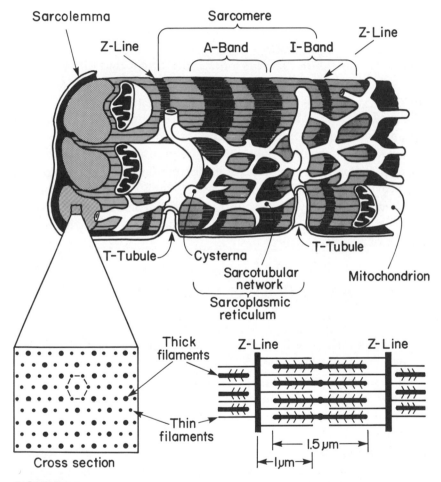

FIGURE 3-1.
Perspective on the organization of myocardial tissue. With lowest magnification (top) myocardial fibers or cells anastamose, forming the *functional syncytium*. The enlargement of an individual cell shows the substructure of that cell with the many sarcomeres lined up in series and parallel. The sarcomere shown below is the functional contractile unit of the myocardial cell and is composed of thick and thin filaments.

Thick filaments are composed primarily of *myosin*. Myosin filaments can be described as having a tail and two heads. The tail is made up of two coiled alpha-helices (fig. 3-2A), and each of the two

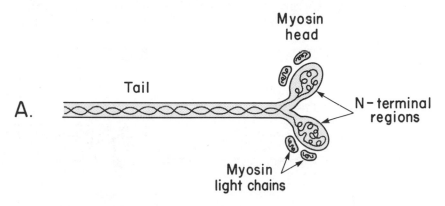

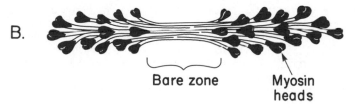

FIGURE 3-2.
Structure of thick filaments. (A) Myosin molecules are made up of two helically entwined polypeptide chains and four light chains. The N-terminal regions of the helical chains (and the associated light chains) form the head of the myosin molecule. (B) Thick filaments are formed when hundreds of these myosin molecules aggregate with their tails close together and their heads arranged at either end of the filament. The heads (which contain the regions of the molecule that split ATP and bind to actin) form the crossbridges between thick and thin filaments.

heads contains the N-terminals of the polypeptide chains of the tail, plus two other polypeptides called *light chains*. Each myosin molecule is therefore made up of six polypeptides: two coiled alpha-helices and four light chains. Thick filaments typically contain hundreds of myosin molecules with the tails packed together and the heads projecting out at both ends of the filament (fig. 3-2B). These heads are the crossbridges that interact with adjacent actin molecules in the sarcomere.

Thin filaments are composed primarily of the protein *actin*. The filaments are double strands of globular subunits twisted into a helix (fig. 3-3). Each globular unit is called *G-actin,* and each chain of G-actin units comprising the double helix is called *F-actin*. Thin filaments contain proteins other than actin as will be described below.

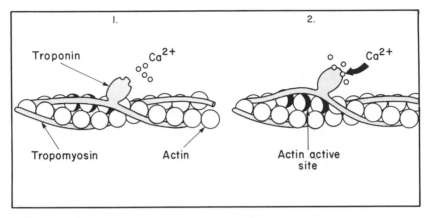

FIGURE 3-3.
Structure of thin filaments. (1) Globular subunits (G-actin) form two strands (F-actin) that twirl around one another. Tropomyosin lies in the grooves formed by the two strands of F-actin. Troponin is attached to tropomyosin at regular intervals. (2) Troponin contains Ca^{2+}-binding sites. When Ca^{2+} becomes bound to troponin, tropomyosin undergoes a conformational change that exposes the actin active site.

Contraction occurs when myosin heads bind to actin filaments and undergo flexion (a conformational change). As the heads flex they pull upon the actin, thus causing the filaments to slide past one another. The flexion of the myosin head requires energy that is supplied by the hydrolysis of ATP (fig. 3-4). Once flexion occurs, the myosin head releases the actin filament. In this way, the thick filaments can be thought of as "walking" along the thin filaments. Because the interactions between different actin and myosin strands occur asynchronously, thin filaments are pulled past thick filaments smoothly.

EXCITATION-CONTRACTION COUPLING

Cardiac muscle fibers contract only when plasma membrane depolarization occurs. Depolarization leads to the initiation of contraction by causing a rise in intracellular Ca^{2+} . When the cardiac fiber

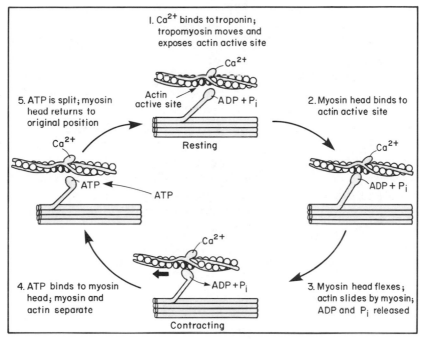

1. Ca^{2+} binds to troponin; tropomyosin moves and exposes actin active site

Ca^{2+}

5. ATP is split; myosin head returns to original position

Actin active site

ADP + P$_i$

Resting

2. Myosin head binds to actin active site

Ca^{2+}

Ca^{2+}

ATP

ATP

ADP + P$_i$

Ca^{2+}

4. ATP binds to myosin head; myosin and actin separate

ADP + P$_i$

Contracting

3. Myosin head flexes; actin slides by myosin; ADP and P$_i$ released

FIGURE 3-4.

Role of Ca^{2+} in myocardial contraction. The addition of Ca^{2+} allows cross-bridge cycling to begin by exposing actin active sites. Myosin heads can then bind to actin and initiate the cycle depicted here. Crossbridge cycling will occur as long as Ca^{2+} and ATP are present. Lack of Ca^{2+} prevents myosin from binding to actin, while lack of ATP prevents myosin from detaching from actin. (P$_i$ = phosphate)

membranes depolarize (as described in chapter 2), Ca^{2+} enters the cells from the extracellular fluid. These ions cause the release of additional Ca^{2+} from sarcoplasmic reticulum within cardiac cells. The Ca^{2+} from the extracellular fluid and sarcoplasmic reticulum raises the Ca^{2+} concentration in the vicinity of the thick and thin filaments. This rise in Ca^{2+} concentration triggers actin-myosin interaction and contraction.

The sensitivity of the actin-myosin interaction to Ca^{2+} depends entirely upon the presence of two regulatory proteins associated with the thin filaments; these are *tropomyosin* and *troponin*. Tropomyosin is a rod-shaped protein that lies in the grooves between the two strands of actin (fig. 3-3), thereby making the thin filament more rigid. Troponin is bound to tropomyosin at specific intervals along the thin filaments. When Ca^{2+} is present, the conformation of troponin changes and it pulls tropomyosin away from a so-called "active" site on the actin molecule (fig. 3-4). This active site can then bind to the myosin head. In this way, a rise in intracellular Ca^{2+} concentration initiates the interaction of actin and myosin.

Myocardial relaxation begins with repolarization (phase 3, fig. 2-1). Relaxation occurs as Ca^{2+} is removed from the cytoplasm by three pathways. First, Ca^{2+} is actively transported into the sarcoplasmic reticulum. Second, it is extruded from the cell in exchange for Na^+, which is subsequently removed by active transport. Finally, it may be taken up by mitochondria in exchange for H^+. As intracellular Ca^{2+} concentration falls, the regulatory proteins once again inhibit the actin-myosin interaction, and relaxation occurs. Various neurotransmitters, hormones, and drugs influence contraction by raising or lowering the concentration of cytoplasmic Ca^{2+} during excitation and/or repolarization, as will be discussed later.

THE CONTRACTION OF ISOLATED CARDIAC MUSCLE

This section examines the contraction of isolated cardiac muscle, and provides an opportunity to explore the basic principles underlying the behavior of the intact heart.

Figure 3-5 shows a conceptual model that has proven to be useful in describing the overall behavior of cardiac muscle. The contractile elements (actin and myosin filaments) are imagined to be arranged in series with various elastic elements, including (1) cell membranes, to which contractile elements are attached; (2) parts of the actin and myosin that stretch during force development; and (3) weaker contractile elements that are pulled apart by stronger ones.[1] When an isolated segment of cardiac muscle is firmly attached at both ends and then stimulated, the ensuing contraction is manifested as an increase in force pulling on the two attachments. The force is generated by the shortening of the contractile elements (actin and myosin sliding past one another) and by the stretching of series elastic elements. The more the contractile elements shorten (and the series elastic stretches), the more force is developed. A contraction with no external shortening of the muscle is called an *isometric contraction*. When the heart contracts with the valves closed, the cardiac muscle undergoes an isometric contraction because no shortening of cardiac muscle fibers occurs. Alternatively, if only one end of the cardiac muscle (fig. 3-5) is fixed and immobile, a load attached to the other end can be lifted (providing the muscle generates a force exceeding the force of gravity on the load). Once

---
[1]Elastic elements arranged in parallel with the contractile elements also exist.

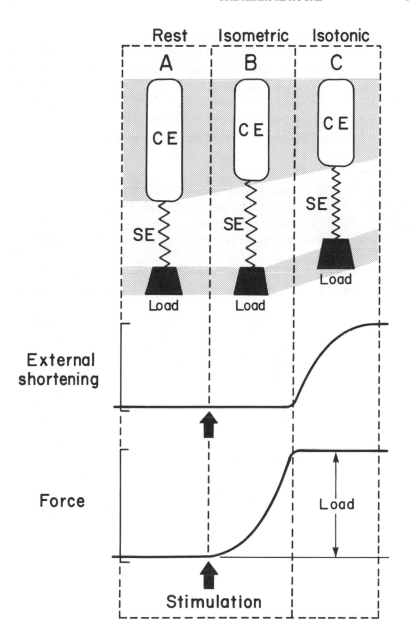

FIGURE 3-5.
Relationship between internal and external shortening and force development. This model of myocardial contraction shows the myocardium at rest in (A). When stimulation occurs, contractile element (CE) shortening begins (B), but until the series elastic element (SE) is stretched enough to develop the force necessary to lift the load, no external shortening occurs. Once the load is lifted (C) no further force development can occur, but shortening begins.

the load is lifted, force development is constant and equal to the force of gravity (i.e., the weight of the load). In this situation the contractile elements shorten with no change in force; this is an *isotonic contraction*. The ventricular muscle contraction that follows the opening of the aortic and pulmonary valves exemplifies a largely isotonic contraction. It is not a perfect example of isotonic contraction because aortic pressure (load) changes during systole.

LENGTH-TENSION RELATIONSHIP

The initial length of cardiac muscle can be adjusted before it is stimulated to contract. Over the range of initial lengths that occur in the intact heart, increased initial length is associated with an increased force development during contraction. However, it is possible to stretch cardiac muscle so much that a decrease in force development results (fig. 3-6). A molecular basis for the relationship is readily apparent (fig. 3-7). As the muscle is stretched, sarcomeres are

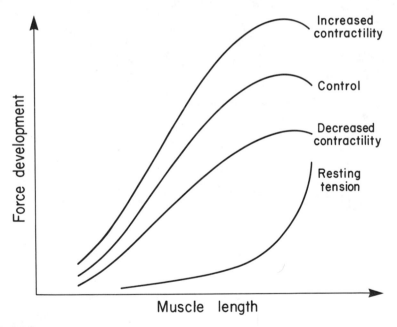

FIGURE 3-6.
Effect of stretching cardiac muscle on force development. Increased length (over a certain range) leads to increased force development. *Contractility* is defined as the force of contraction at a given length; therefore, increased contractility means increased force of contraction at a given length. The passive resting tension caused by stretching the muscle begins to increase dramatically at the point where further length increases do not cause further increases in active force development.

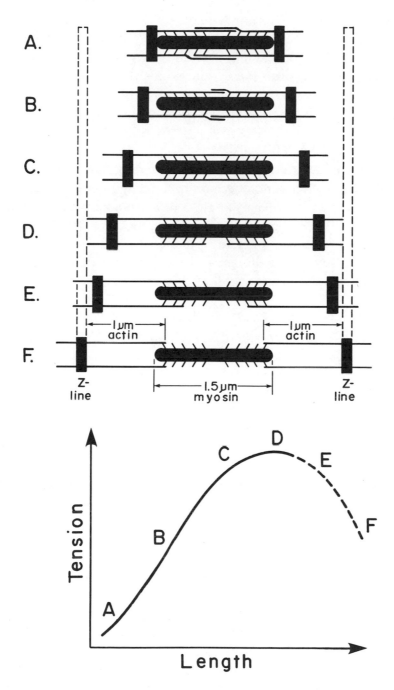

FIGURE 3-7.
Molecular basis for the length-tension relationship of muscle.

progressively lengthened until a perfect overlap between the active sites of actin and the myosin heads occurs. Further stretching reduces the number of matching sites and decreases the force development. This is the main, but not the exclusive, explanation for the relationship between initial length and force of contraction. Other factors involve changes in the concentration of cytosolic Ca^{2+}.

PRELOAD AND AFTERLOAD

The load stretching a resting muscle is called the *preload*. It determines force of contraction because of the length-tension relationship just described. When a muscle contracts under the conditions shown in fig. 3-5, the load that is lifted (in panel C) is the *afterload*; that is, the load is not apparent to the muscle until after it begins shortening. The heart behaves as an afterloaded muscle because it experiences aortic pressure only after the aortic valve opens.

FORCE-VELOCITY RELATIONSHIP

When cardiac muscle is stimulated to contract against a variety of loads, it becomes evident that shortening occurs more quickly if the load (afterload) is light and the force development is small, and more slowly if the load is heavy. In an isometric contraction there is a velocity of shortening of zero, since no shortening occurs. Alternatively, with zero external load, shortening velocity is maximal (V_{max}, fig. 3-8A). Norepinephrine can increase the force of contraction for a particular velocity of shortening. Other agents, as well as increased length and heart rate, also have this effect. The relationship between the strength and speed of contraction is the *force-velocity relationship*.

CONTRACTILITY

Norepinephrine has three effects on the isometric contraction of cardiac muscle: these are (1) increased peak force of contraction, (2) increased rate of force development, and (3) increased rate of relaxation. If an isotonic (instead of an isometric) contraction is studied, norepinephrine causes an increase in the peak shortening, velocity of shortening, and rate of relaxation. A change in peak force development or shortening at a particular initial length is defined as a change in *contractility*. The increase in peak force and shortening (in response to norepinephrine) occurs with any given initial length

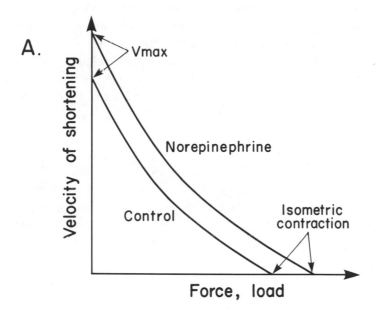

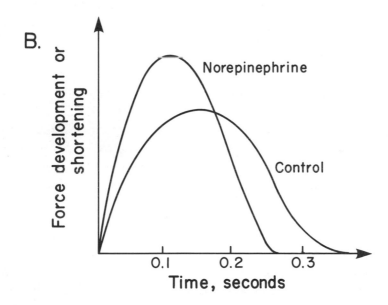

FIGURE 3-8.
Effect of norepinephrine on myocardial contraction. Norepinephrine causes increased contractility of cardiac muscle. This is manifested as a greater velocity of shortening at a given force development (A) and an increase in shortening or force development at a fixed initial length (B).

and therefore is an example of an increase in contractility. The increase in force of contraction that occurs when muscle is stretched (fig. 3-7) is *not* an example of increased contractility because no increase in contractile force occurs for a given muscle length. Figure 3-8 shows that increased contractility can also be viewed as an increase in the velocity of shortening for a particular degree of afterload.

At the level of the contractile proteins, two factors are responsible for increasing contractility. The first is an accelerated rate of crossbridge cycling; that is, the cycle of myosin head attachment to actin, head flexion, and detachment from actin occurs more quickly. The faster crossbridge cycling results in an increased velocity of shortening. The second factor is an increase in the number of actin-myosin crossbridge attachments, resulting in more force development. The cause of the increased number of crossbridge attachments is better understood than the cause of the faster rate of crossbridge cycling. The increased number of crossbridge attachments results from the higher levels of cytosolic Ca^{2+}. As more troponin molecules are bound to the Ca^{2+}, additional actin active sites are exposed. This enables more myosin heads to attach to actin, which raises peak force development. The faster rate of crossbridge cycling probably relates to a modification of the myosin head resulting from its phosphorylation by a protein kinase.

Many of the effects of norepinephrine can be linked to a rise in cellular *cyclic adenosine monophosphate (cAMP)*. Elevated cAMP causes activation of several protein kinases, which results in the phosphorylation of at least three important proteins: (1) the myosin head, (2) a sarcoplasmic reticulum membrane protein regulating Ca^{2+} uptake, and (3) a plasma membrane protein controlling slow Ca^{2+} channels (fig. 3-9). Myosin head phosphorylation may be responsible for the increased rate of crossbridge cycling. Phosphorylation of the sarcoplasmic reticulum protein stimulates the active transport of Ca^{2+} into the sarcoplasmic reticulum, producing two effects. First, it increases the rate of relaxation by causing cytosolic Ca^{2+} to fall more rapidly. Second, it builds up the sarcoplasmic reticulum content of Ca^{2+} so that more can be released during excitation. This contributes to a higher cytosolic Ca^{2+} concentration, which in turn raises peak force development. Finally, phosphorylation of a specific plasma membrane protein causes more Ca^{2+} to enter the cytosol across the plasma membrane via the slow calcium

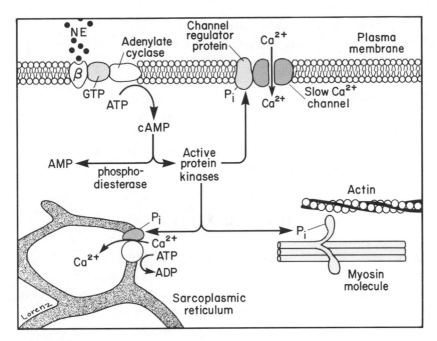

FIGURE 3-9.

Intracellular changes produced by norepinephrine. Norepinephrine binds to a plasma membrane receptor (β-receptor) that (via the GTP-binding protein) activates adenylate cyclase. The resulting increase in cAMP activates *protein kinases* that phosphorylate (1) proteins in the plasma membrane and sarcoplasmic reticulum and (2) the myosin head. The result is increased Ca^{2+} entry via slow channels, increased Ca^{2+} pumping by sarcoplasmic reticulum, and increased rate of crossbridge cycling. The net effect on cytosol Ca^{2+} is to increase its peak concentration during excitation and to accelerate its rate of rise and fall at the beginning and end of excitation. cAMP is degraded to AMP by phosphodiesterase. The site of phosphorylation on the myosin head shown here is distinct from the site responsible for ATPase activity (fig. 3-4). Guanosine triphosphate (GTP) is necessary for the activation of adenylate cyclase. (P_i — phosphate)

channels, which also raises cytosolic Ca^{2+} concentration and promotes force development.

Certain cardiac drugs influence contractility by affecting the concentration of cytoplasmic Ca^{2+} during excitation and/or repolarization. For example, cardiac glycosides (digitalis or digoxin) are used to strengthen the force of contraction in failing hearts. The usefulness of digitalis in the setting of heart failure stems from its ability to raise intracellular Ca^{2+} by partially inhibiting the Na^+, K^+ ATPase in the cell membrane (fig. 2-2). This causes the concentration of cytoplasmic Na^+ to rise and reduces the gradient that normally drives Na^+ into the cell. The decline in Na^+ entry subsequently slows the rate of Ca^{2+} extrusion from the cytosol ($Na^+ - Ca^{2+}$ exchange; see fig. 2-2). In contrast, drugs called *calcium entry blockers* (of which verapamil and diltiazem are examples) are used clinically to attenuate myocardial contractility. This action is valuable in situations where it is desirable to minimize the work of the heart, for example, when myocardial blood flow is severely limited by coronary artery stenosis or other conditions. As the name implies, these drugs act by blocking the channels in the cell membrane through which Ca^{2+} normally enters.

THE CARDIAC CYCLE

Now consider the way in which cyclic contractions of cardiac muscle cause the heart to pump blood. The cycle of events described here occurs almost simultaneously in the right and left hearts; the main difference is that the pressures are higher on the left side. Discussions will be limited to the events occurring in the left side of the heart. The P wave reflects atrial depolarization, which initiates *atrial systole*. Contraction of the atrium "tops off" ventricular filling with a final small volume of blood from the atria. Atrial systole is not essential for ventricular filling, and in its absence ventricular filling is only slightly reduced. The P wave is followed by an electrically quiet period during which AV node transmission occurs (PR interval).

The QRS complex reflects excitation of ventricular muscle and the beginning of ventricular systole (fig. 3-10). As ventricular pressure rises above atrial pressure, the mitral valve closes. Contraction of the papillary muscles keeps the mitral valve from everting into the left atrium and enables the valve to prevent the regurgitation of blood into the atrium as pressure rises. The aortic valve does not open until left ventricular pressure exceeds aortic pressure. During the interval when both mitral and aortic valves are closed, the ventricular muscle contracts isometrically because ventricular volume cannot change. Instead, the contraction causes ventricular pressure to rise. As ventricular pressure exceeds aortic pressure (at approximately 80 mmHg), the aortic valve opens and allows blood to flow from the ventricle into the aorta. Ventricular muscle begins to shorten, reducing the volume of the ventricle. As the rate of ejection begins to fall (see the aortic flow record), the aortic and ventricular

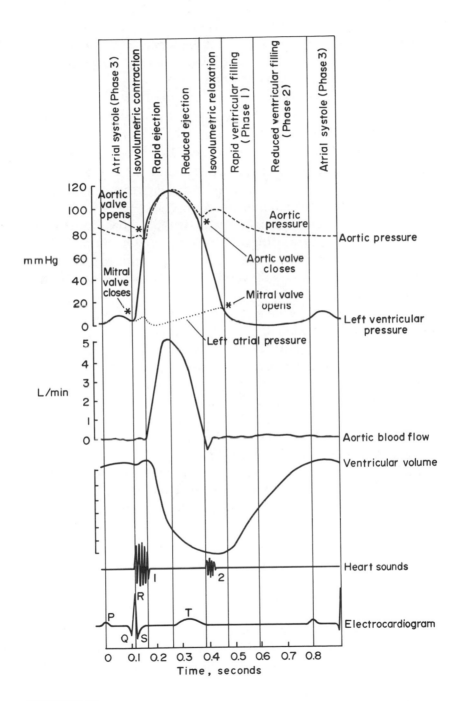

FIGURE 3-10.
Timing of various events within the cardiac cycle.

pressures decline. Ventricular pressure actually decreases below aortic pressure prior to the closure of the aortic valve, but flow continues through the aortic valve because of inertia imparted to the blood by ventricular contraction.[2]

Ventricular repolarization (producing the T wave) initiates ventricular relaxation, and as the ventricular pressure drops below atrial pressure the mitral valve opens. This allows the blood accumulated within the atrium during ventricular systole to flow rapidly into the ventricle, initiating the first phase of ventricular filling. Both pressures continue to decrease—the atrial pressure because of emptying into the ventricle, and the ventricular pressure because of continued ventricular relaxation (which in turn draws more blood from the atrium). Midway through the *ventricular diastole*, filling slows as ventricular and atrial pressures become equal (second phase). Atrial systole tops off ventricular volume during the third phase of ventricular filling.

Ventricular diastole and systole can be thought of in terms of either electrical or mechanical events. Electrically, ventricular systole is defined as the period between the QRS complex and the end of the T wave. Mechanically, ventricular systole is the period between the closure of the mitral valve and the subsequent closure of the aortic valve. In either case ventricular diastole comprises the remainder of the cycle. The *first (S₁)* and *second (S₂)* heart sounds signal the beginning and end of mechanical systole. The first heart sound (usually described by the physician as a "lub") occurs as the ventricle contracts and ventricular pressure rises above atrial pressure (fig. 3-11). This causes the atrioventricular valves to close, producing a relatively low-pitched sound. In contrast, the aortic and pulmonary valves close at the end of ventricular systole, when the ventricles relax and pressure in the ventricle diminishes below that in the arteries. This produces the second heart sound, which is relatively high-pitched (typically described as a "dup"). Mechanical events other than the closure of the valves probably contribute to these two sounds, especially S1. These factors include movement of the great vessels and heart walls, and turbulence of the rapidly moving blood. The third and fourth heart sounds are also caused by these factors, but these are usually inaudible in normally functioning hearts.

---

[2]If that gives you trouble, think of a rubber ball connected to a paddle by a rubber band. The ball continues to travel away from the paddle after you pull back because the inertial force on the ball exceeds the force generated by the rubber band.

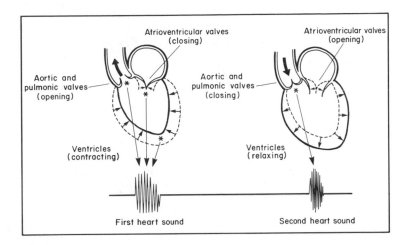

FIGURE 3-11.
Production of the heart sounds. The curve traces the sounds heard with closure of the atrioventricular valves (first heart sound) and the aortic and pulmonary valves (second heart sound). Turbulent blood flow and ventricular
wall motion may contribute to the heart sounds, especially the first. The second heart sound is often heard as a distinct first component (aortic valve closure) and second component (pulmonary valve closure); this so-called
"splitting" usually widens with inspiration and may disappear with expiration.

CARDIAC OUTPUT

Cardiac output is defined as the volume of blood ejected from the
heart per unit time. The usual resting values quoted for adult humans range from 5 to 6 L/min, or approximately 8% of the body
weight per minute.[3] Cardiac output is the product of heart rate and
stroke volume (the volume of blood ejected with each beat). If
heart rate remains constant, cardiac output increases in proportion
to the stroke volume, and vice versa. Table 3-1 outlines the factors
that influence cardiac output.

FACTORS INFLUENCING CARDIAC OUTPUT
Stroke Volume
Stroke volume is determined by the balance between force of contraction and afterload. The factors that determine force of contraction will be discussed first.

---

[3]Cardiac output divided by body surface area is called the *cardiac index*. When some sort of normal-
ization is necessary to compare the cardiac output among individuals of different sizes, either cardiac
index or the cardiac output divided by body weight can be used.

Table 3-1.

Factors Influencing Cardiac Output

I. Stroke volume
  A. Force of contraction
    1. End diastolic fiber length (heterometric autoregulation, Starling's law, ventricular function curves, preload)
    2. Contractility
      a. Sympathetic stimulation with norepinephrine (and epinephrine); mediated via β-receptor
      b. Drugs (digitalis, anesthetics, toxins, etc.)
      c. Disease (coronary artery disease, myocarditis, etc.)
      d. Homeometric autoregulation
    3. Hypertrophy
  B. Afterload
    1. Ventricular radius
    2. Aortic pressure

II. Heart rate (and pattern of electrical excitation)

FORCE OF CONTRACTION

The amount of blood ejected from the ventricle during systole is dependent upon the force with which the myocardium contracts. As table 3-1 shows, the factors that determine force of contraction are end diastolic fiber length, contractility, and hypertrophy.

End Diastolic Fiber Length

The relationship between ventricular end diastolic fiber length (preload) and stroke volume is known as Starling's law of the heart, or *heterometric autoregulation*. Within limits, increases in the left ventricular end diastolic fiber length augment the ventricular force of contraction, which increases the stroke volume. This reflects the relationship between muscle length and force of contraction shown in fig. 3-6. After reaching an optimal diastolic fiber length, stroke volume begins to decrease with further stretching of the ventricle (fig. 3-12).

End diastolic fiber length is determined by the end diastolic volume, which in turn is dependent upon the end diastolic pressure. For a given ventricular *compliance* (change in volume caused by a given change in pressure), higher end diastolic pressures increase both the diastolic volume and the fiber length. Furthermore, the end diastolic pressure depends upon the degree of ventricular filling that occurs during ventricular diastole, which is influenced largely by the atrial pressure. Thus the curve in fig. 3-12 is often plotted

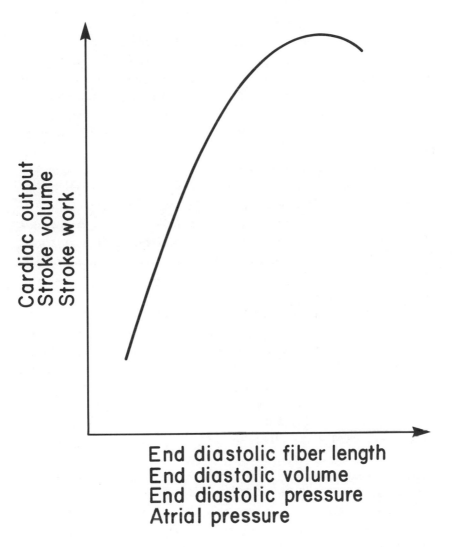

FIGURE 3-12.
Ventricular function curve. Several combinations of variables can be used to plot the ventricular response curve.

with either end diastolic volume, end diastolic pressure, or atrial pressure as the abscissa rather than end diastolic fiber length.

The ordinate on the plot of Starling's law of the heart (fig. 3-12) can also be a variable other than stroke volume. For example, if heart rate remains constant, cardiac output can be substituted for stroke volume. The effect of mean arterial pressure on stroke volume should also be taken into account, since an increase in mean arterial

pressure decreases stroke volume by increasing the force that opposes the ejection of blood during systole (afterload). To correct for
this, stroke volume times mean arterial pressure is often plotted on
the ordinate instead of stroke volume alone. Fortunately, the mean
arterial pressure multiplied by the stroke volume is a good approximation of the external work of the heart; this is called the *stroke
work*. If stroke work is on the ordinate, any increase in the force of
contraction that results in an increase in pressure (rather than an increase in stroke volume) shifts the stroke work curve upward and to
the left. If stroke volume were the dependent variable, no change in
the performance of the heart would be expressed by the curve.

Any combination of these variables is called a *ventricular function curve,* and it expresses Starling's law of the heart. This relationship is also called heterometric autoregulation because it is intrinsic
to the heart (autoregulation) and is elicited by changes in ventricular fiber length (heterometric).

Starling's law of the heart (i.e., ventricular function curves or
heterometric autoregulation) helps to solve the difficult problem of
balancing the output between the two ventricles. If the right heart
were to pump 1% more blood than the left heart per minute without
a compensatory mechanism, the entire blood volume of the body
would be displaced into the pulmonary circulation in less than two
hours. On the other hand, a similar error in the opposite direction
would likewise displace all the blood volume into the systemic circuit. Fortunately, heterometric autoregulation prevents this. If the
right ventricle pumps slightly more blood than the left ventricle, left
atrial filling (and pressure) will increase. As left atrial pressure increases, left ventricular pressure and left ventricular end diastolic
fiber length increase both the force of contraction and the stroke
volume of the left ventricle. If the stroke volume rises too much, the
left heart begins to pump more blood than the right heart and left
atrial pressure drops; this decreases left ventricular filling and reduces stroke volume. The process continues until the left heart output is exactly equal to the right heart output (fig. 3-13).

The descending limb of the ventricular function curve,
analogous to the descending limb of the length/force curve (fig. 3-
6), is probably never reached in the normal heart because the resistance to stretch increases as the end diastolic volume begins to
exceed the limits for optimum stroke volume. The increased resistance to stretch *(decreased compliance)* means that atrial pressures

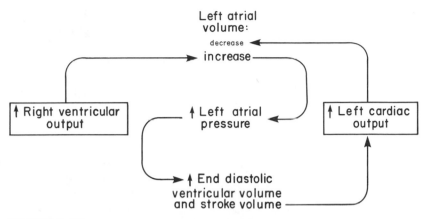

FIGURE 3-13.
Starling's law and cardiac output. The diagram demonstrates how Starling's law keeps the output of the left and right hearts balanced. Heart rate is assumed to be constant.

necessary to produce further filling of the ventricle are seldom (if ever) reached. The limited compliance therefore prevents optimal sarcomere length from being exceeded. Should the heart fail due to a disease process, it can dilate beyond this normal limit because it becomes less resistant to stretch (*increased compliance*). However, even under these conditions, it is likely that optimal sarcomere length will not be exceeded. Instead, the sarcomeres appear to slip past each other, allowing the muscle to lengthen without exceeding the optimal sarcomere length.

Contractility

Factors other than the end diastolic fiber length can influence the force of ventricular contraction, and there is a family of curves relating stroke volume (or work) to end diastolic fiber length under different conditions. For example, increases in sympathetic nerve activity increase the force of contraction for a given end diastolic fiber length (fig. 3-14). The increased force of contraction causes more blood to be ejected against a given aortic pressure and thus raises stroke volume. A change in the force of contraction at a constant end diastolic fiber length reflects a change in the contractility of the heart. A shift in the ventricular function curve to the left indicates increased contractility (i.e., more force and/or shortening occur at the same initial fiber length), and shifts to the right indicate decreased contractility. In some instances an increase in contractility will be accompanied by an increase in arterial pressure. If this occurs, the stroke volume may remain constant, and the increased

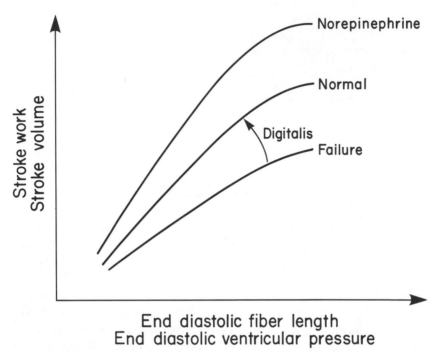

FIGURE 3-14.
Effect of norepinephrine and heart failure on the ventricular function curve.

contractility will not be evident by plotting the stroke volume against the end diastolic fiber length. Instead, if stroke work is plotted, a leftward shift of the ventricular curve will be observed (fig. 3-14). A ventricular function curve with stroke volume on the ordinate can be used only to indicate changes in contractility when arterial pressure does not change.

During heart failure, the ventricular function curve is shifted to the right, causing a particular end diastolic fiber length to be associated with less force of contraction and/or shortening, and a smaller stroke volume. As previously described, cardiac glycosides tend to restore contractility to normal: that is, they shift the ventricular curve of the failing heart back to the left (fig. 3-14).

Another influence on contractility is homeometric autoregulation, discussed in the subsequent section on aortic pressure.

Hypertrophy
The force of contraction is also increased by *myocardial hypertrophy*. Repeated bouts of increased cardiac output (as occurs with

physical exercise) or a sustained elevation of arterial pressure results in increased synthesis of contractile proteins and enlargement of cardiac myocytes. As each cell enlarges, the ventricular wall thickens and is capable of greater force development.

In summary, the force of contraction can be influenced in three ways. The first way includes those events that alter end diastolic fiber length and thereby change the force of contraction (as expressed by a particular ventricular function curve). The second way includes events that change contractility (and shift a given ventricular function curve), such as exposure to norepinephrine, drugs, and homeometric autoregulation. The third way involves hypertrophy of the myocardium (table 3-1).

AFTERLOAD

In addition to force of contraction, stroke volume is influenced by the afterload against which the ventricle must shorten to eject blood. Afterload is determined by ventricular radius and aortic pressure.

Ventricular Radius

The ventricular radius influences stroke volume because of the relationship between ventricular pressures (P_v) and ventricular wall tension (T). For a hollow structure, it is expressed by the LaPlace equation:

$$P_v = T\left(\frac{1}{r_1} + \frac{1}{r_2}\right)$$

where r_1 and r_2 are the radii of curvature for the ventricular wall. Figure 3-15 shows this relationship for a simpler structure in which

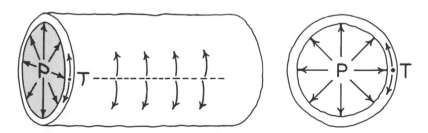

FIGURE 3-15.
Pressure and tension in a cylindrical blood vessel. The tension is a force tending to open an imaginary slit along the length of the blood vessel.

curvature occurs in only one dimension (i.e., a cylinder). In this case r_2 approaches ∞. Therefore:

$$P_v = T\left(\frac{1}{r_1}\right) \text{ or } T = P_v r_1.$$

The internal pressure expands the cylinder until it is exactly balanced by the wall tension. The larger the radius, the larger the tension needed to balance a particular pressure. Almost everyone has partially inflated a long balloon so that there is an inflated part with a large radius and an uninflated part with a much smaller radius. The pressure inside the balloon is the same everywhere, yet the tension in the wall is much higher in the inflated part because the radius is much greater (fig. 3-16).

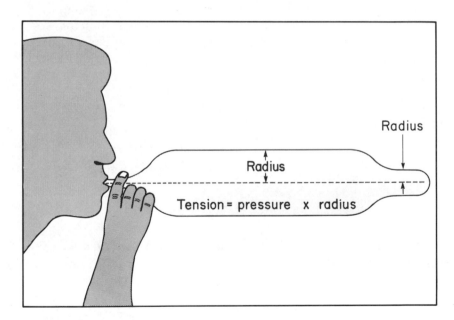

FIGURE 3-16.
Effect of cylinder radius on tension. In a balloon the tension in the wall is proportional to the radius since the pressure is the same everywhere inside the balloon.

These general principles also apply to noncylindrical objects such as the heart and the tapering blood vessels. When the ventricular chamber enlarges, the wall tension required to balance a given intraventricular pressure increases. As a result, the force required for ventricular contraction likewise increases with ventricular size.

Within physiological limits, an increase in ventricular size raises both wall tension and stroke volume. This occurs because the positive effects of adjustment in sarcomere length overcompensate for the negative effects of increasing ventricular radius. However, if a ventricle becomes pathologically dilated, the myocardial fibers may be unable to generate enough tension to raise pressure to the normal systolic level, and the stroke volume may fall.

Aortic Pressure

The second determinant of afterload is the aortic pressure. If arterial pressure is suddenly increased, a ventricular contraction (at a given level of contractility and end diastolic fiber length) produces a lower stroke volume. This decrease can be predicted from the force-velocity relationship of cardiac muscle (fig. 3-8). The shortening velocity of ventricular muscle decreases with increasing load, and for a given duration of contraction (reflecting the given duration of the action potential) the lower velocity results in less shortening and a decreased stroke volume (fig. 3-17). This causes the left ventricle to eject less blood per beat, although the output from the right heart remains constant. Left ventricular filling subsequently exceeds its output. As the end diastolic volume and fiber length of the left ventricle increase, the ventricular force of contraction is enhanced. A new steady state is quickly reached in which the end diastolic fiber length is increased, and the previous stroke volume is maintained.

Within limits, however, additional compensations occur. Over the next 30 seconds, the end diastolic fiber length returns toward the control level, while the stroke volume is maintained despite the increase in aortic pressure. If arterial pressure times stroke volume (stroke work) is plotted against end diastolic fiber length, it is apparent that stroke work has increased for a given end diastolic fiber length. This leftward shift of the ventricular function curve indicates an increase in contractility. Because there is a change in the force of contraction occurring independently of end diastolic fiber length, this phenomenon is called *homeometric autoregulation* (same length self-regulation). Homeometric autoregulation is a relatively minor influence, however, and causes a small increase in contractility compared with that produced by an increase in sympathetic nerve activity.

Heart Rate

Heart rate varies from under 50 beats per minute in a resting, physically fit individual to over 200 beats per minute during maximal ex-

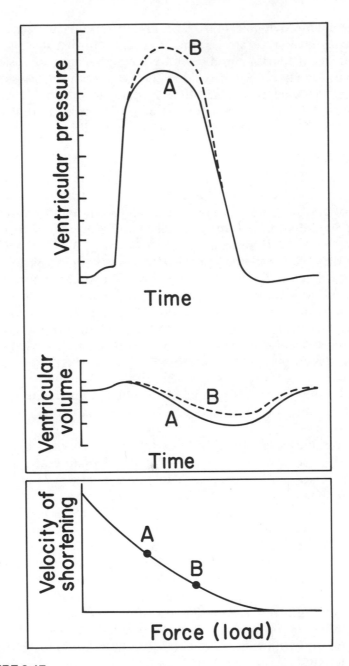

FIGURE 3-17.
Effect of aortic pressure on ventricular function. Ventricular pressure, ventricular volume, and force-velocity relationship are shown for normal (A) and elevated (B) aortic pressure. The slower velocity of shortening means less ventricular emptying and a lower stroke volume.

ercise. If stroke volume is held constant, increases in heart rate cause proportional increases in cardiac output. Normally, more than half of the rise in cardiac output produced by strenuous exercise is due to increased heart rate. In contrast, decreases in heart rate (due to stimulation of the cardiac parasympathetic nerves or other causes) reduce cardiac output very little. As the heart rate falls, the end diastolic fiber length of the ventricles increases; this occurs because the longer duration of diastole results in greater filling. The elevated end diastolic fiber length increases stroke volume, which compensates for the decreased heart rate. This balance works until the heart rate is below 20, at which point additional increases in end diastolic fiber length cannot augment stroke volume further because the peak of the ventricular function curve has been reached.

The effects of increased heart rate are analogous, but more complex. If an electronic pacemaker is attached to the right atrium and the heart rate is increased by electrical stimulation, surprisingly little increase in cardiac output results. As the heart rate increases, the interval between beats shortens and the duration of diastole decreases. The decrease in diastole leaves less time for ventricular filling, producing a shortened end diastolic fiber length; this subsequently reduces both the force of contraction and the stroke volume. The increased heart rate is therefore offset by the decrease in stroke volume. Events within the myocardium compensate to some degree for the decreased time available for filling. First, increases in the heart rate reduce the duration of the action potential, and thus the duration of systole, which increases the time available for diastolic filling. In addition, faster heart rates are accompanied by an increase in the force of contraction, which tends to maintain stroke volume. The increased contractility is sometimes called *treppe* or the *staircase phenomenon*. It is classified under the heading of homeometric autoregulation because the increase in contractile force occurs at a constant end diastolic fiber length. These internal adjustments are not very effective, and by themselves would be insufficient to permit heart rate to play a predominant role in the control of cardiac output. However, increased heart rate usually occurs because of decreased parasympathetic and increased sympathetic neural activity. The release of norepinephrine by sympathetic nerves not only increases the heart rate as described in chapter 2, but also dramatically increases the force of contraction (fig. 3-14). Furthermore, norepinephrine increases conduction velocity in the heart, which results in a more efficient and rapid ejection of blood from the ventricles. These effects, summarized in fig. 3-18, maintain the stroke volume as heart rate increases. Thus when heart rate increases physiologically due to an increase in sympathetic nervous system activity (as during exercise), cardiac output increases proportionately over a broad range.

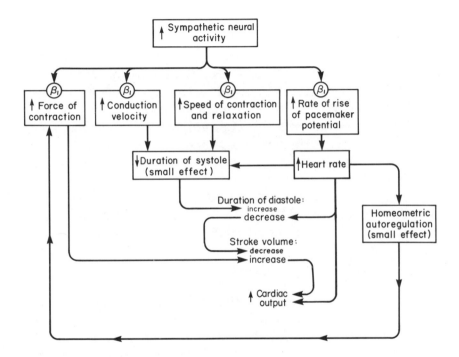

FIGURE 3-18.
Effects of increased sympathetic neural activity on heart rate, stroke volume, and cardiac output. Various effects of norepinephrine on the heart compensate for the decreased duration of diastole and hold stroke volume relatively constant so that cardiac output increases with increasing heart rate.

Without the increased contractility caused by norepinephrine, the elevation in heart rate would produce very little increase in cardiac output. For example, when the rate increases above 180 beats per minute secondary to an abnormal pacemaker, stroke volume begins to fall because of poor diastolic filling and inadequate myocardial contractility. A person with tachycardia (caused, for example, by an ectopic ventricular pacemaker) may therefore have a reduction in cardiac output despite an increased rate.

SUMMARY OF DETERMINANTS OF CARDIAC OUTPUT

Stroke volume can be affected by changing the contractile force of the ventricular myocardium or by changing the force opposing ejection (the aortic pressure or afterload). The contractile force depends upon (1) the ventricular end diastolic fiber length (Starling's law) and (2) the myocardial contractility. Contractility is influenced by four major factors: (1) norepinephrine release from sympathetic nerves and to a lesser extent norepinephrine and epinephrine release from the adrenal medulla; (2) certain hormones and drugs including glucagon, isoproterenol, digitalis (increasing contractility), and anesthetics (decreasing contractility); (3) disease states, for example, coronary artery disease, myocarditis, bacterial toxins, alterations in plasma electrolytes, and acid-base balance; and (4) homeometric autoregulation, which includes (a) increased contractility with increased heart rate and (b) increased myocardial contractility with increased mean arterial pressure. Changes in heart rate also play a major role in determining cardiac output.

MEASUREMENT OF CARDIAC OUTPUT

Cardiac output can be measured using variations of the Fick principle (Fick's law), which is based upon the conservation of mass. The application of this principle is best understood by considering the measurement of a volume of blood in a beaker (fig. 3-19). If the beaker contains an unknown volume of blood, the volume could be determined by dispersing a known quantity of dye throughout it, and then measuring the concentration of dye in a sample of blood. The quantity of dye (known) in the blood is equal to the concentration of dye in the blood (measured) times the volume of blood (unknown):

Quantity of dye (A) = Concentration of dye (C) × volume of blood (V). This is a rearranged version of the definition of concentration:

$$C = A/V \text{ and } V = A/C$$

In the case of cardiac output, the goal is to measure the volume of blood flowing through the heart per unit of time.

If all the cardiac output were to be trapped in a beaker for one minute, and a known quantity of dye was added to it, the cardiac output could be computed according to the above calculations. This is, of course, impractical because (1) the volume in the beaker can be measured directly, and (2) the subject might exsanguinate.

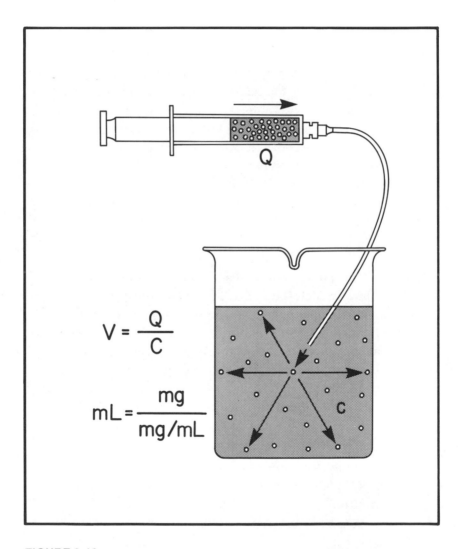

FIGURE 3-19.
Measurement of volume by the dye dilution method. The volume (V) of fluid in the beaker equals the quantity (Q) of dye divided by the concentration (C) of the dye dispersed in the liquid.

When the *dye* or *indicator dilution method* is used, a known quantity of dye can be injected into the circulation, and the blood downstream can be serially sampled after the dye has had a chance to mix (fig. 3-20). The dye is injected on the venous side of the circulation, and the sampling is performed from a distal arterial vessel.

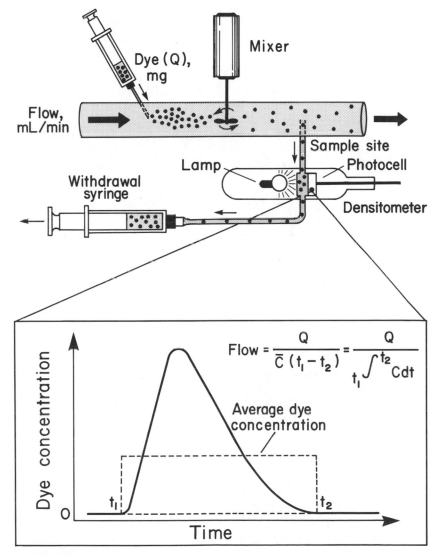

FIGURE 3-20.
Dye dilution method for determining flow through a tube. The volume per minute flowing in the tube equals the quantity of dye injected divided by the average dye concentration ($\overline{C}$) at the sample site, multiplied by the time between the appearance (t_1) and disappearance (t_2) of the dye.

The resulting concentration of dye in the distal arterial blood (C) will change with time (fig. 3-21). First the concentration rises as those dye particles carried by the fastest moving blood reach the arterial sampling point. Concentration rises to a peak as the majority of the dye particles arrive and then falls off as the slower ones get there.

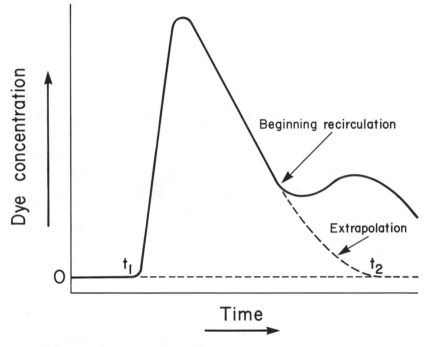

FIGURE 3-21.
Effect of recirculation on the dye concentration curve. Recirculation of dye prevents direct use of the concentration curves in calculation of cardiac output. The initial part of the curve is extrapolated to get an estimate of the true dye concentration curve.

Before the slowest ones arrive, the fastest come around again via the shortest pathways (recirculation). The method for dealing with the recirculation is described later. Assuming no recirculation (as in Fig. 3-20), the average concentration of dye can be determined. To do this, one measures the dye concentration continuously from its first appearance (t_1) until its disappearance (t_2). The average concentration ($\overline{C}$) over that period is determined and:

$$\text{cardiac output} = \dot{Q} = A/_{t_1}\!\int^{t_2} \overline{C}\,dt = A/\overline{C} \times [t_1 - t_2]).$$

Note the similarity between this equation and the equation for calculating volume in a beaker. On the left-hand side is a volume per minute (rather than a volume); on the right-hand side is an amount of dye in the numerator, while in the denominator is the product of concentration and time (rather than a concentration). Concentration, volume, and amount appear in this equation (as in the previous equation), but time is present in the denominator on both sides.

Before the entire arterial concentration curve needed to calculate the average concentration can be obtained the dye begins to recirculate, giving a falsely high value for the arterial concentration (fig. 3-21). To correct for this, the downslope of the curve is assumed to be semilogarithmic and the arterial value is extrapolated. The above method is called the dye or indicator dilution method.

Another way in which the conservation of mass is used to calculate cardiac output involves the continuous entry of oxygen into the blood via the lungs (fig. 3-22). In a steady state, the oxygen leaving the lungs per minute via the pulmonary veins must equal the oxygen entering the lungs via (1) the (mixed) venous blood and (2) respiration (in a steady state, the amount of oxygen replaced by respiration

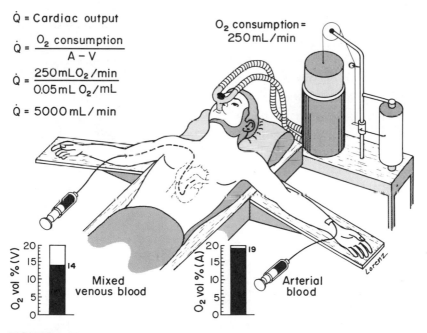

$\dot{Q}$ = Cardiac output

$$\dot{Q} = \frac{O_2 \text{ consumption}}{A - V}$$

$$\dot{Q} = \frac{250\,mL\,O_2/min}{0.05\,mL\,O_2/mL}$$

$\dot{Q}$ = 5000 mL/min

O_2 consumption = 250 mL/min

Mixed venous blood

Arterial blood

FIGURE 3-22.
Calculation of cardiac output using the Fick principle.

is equal to the amount consumed by body metabolism):

$$O_2\,(\text{out}) = O_2\,(\text{in})$$

or:

pulmonary vein O_2 output = pulmonary artery (mixed venous) O_2 input + O_2 added by respiration (equal to O_2 consumption).

The pulmonary vein O_2 output is also equal to the pulmonary vein oxygen content (same as arterial O_2 content, or AO_2) multiplied by the cardiac output ($\dot{Q}$). Mixed venous O_2 input is likewise defined as mixed venous O_2 content (VO_2) multiplied by cardiac output. Using $\dot{V}O_2$ for oxygen consumption, it follows by substitution that:

$$\dot{Q} \times AO_2 = (\dot{Q} \times VO_2) + \dot{V}O_2$$

which rearranges to:

$$\dot{Q} = \frac{\dot{V}O_2}{AO_2 - VO_2}$$

Systemic arterial blood O_2 content, pulmonary arterial (mixed venous) blood O_2 content, and oxygen consumption can all be measured, therefore cardiac output can be calculated. The theory for this method is more sound than that for the dye dilution method because it avoids the need for extrapolation. However, the avoidance of cardiac catheterization required to measure pulmonary artery oxygen content makes the dye dilution method the more popular one. The two methods agree very well in a wide variety of circumstances.

In most clinical situations, cardiac output is measured using a variation of the dye dilution method called *thermodilution.* A *Swan-Ganz* catheter is placed into a large vein and threaded through the right atrium and ventricle so that its tip lies in the pulmonary artery. The catheter is designed so that a known amount of ice-cold saline solution can be injected into the right side of the heart via a sideport in the catheter. This solution decreases the temperature of the surrounding blood. The magnitude of the fall in temperature depends upon the volume of blood that mixes with the solution, which in turn depends upon the cardiac output. A thermistor on the catheter tip (located downstream in the pulmonary artery) measures the fall in blood temperature. Using calculations similar to those described for the dye dilution method, one can determine the cardiac output.

ENERGETICS OF CARDIAC FUNCTION

The heart takes chemical energy in the form of ATP and converts it into mechanical work and heat. The external mechanical work per beat *(stroke work, SW)* can be calculated as the mean ventricular systolic pressure $(\overline{P_v})$ multiplied by the volume moved, or *stroke volume (SV)*: $SW = P_v \times SV$. This is analogous to lifting a weight a certain distance and calculating the mechanical work as the force times the distance. Although there is a difference between the mean arterial pressure $(\overline{P_a})$ and the mean ventricular systolic pressure, mean arterial pressure is usually used as an approximation to calculate external work:

$$SW = \overline{P}_a \times SV$$

Since the total energy used by the heart can be calculated from the oxygen consumed, the efficiency of the heart in performing work can be measured. Only 3% (approximately) of the energy liberated from oxygen is used for external work under resting conditions. This percentage varies threefold or fourfold under different conditions, and therefore changes in external work do not tell us much about changes in energy consumption of the heart. This occurs because most of the energy not lost directly as heat is used to maintain the force of the contraction (and thus the ventricular pressure) rather than to eject the blood. The importance of this can be seen by comparing two tasks: in one case, lifting a 20-lb weight from the floor to a table; in the other case, lifting the weight to the table height and continuing to hold it. The second task is clearly more difficult, even though the external work done (i.e., the force times the distance that the object was moved) in each case is the same. The ventricles not only develop the pressure required to move the blood, but must hold the pressure during systole. The maintenance of pressure takes far more energy than the external work alone as calculated from ventricular pressure and stroke volume. In fact, if the external work of the heart is raised by increasing the stroke volume, but not the mean arterial pressure, the oxygen consumption of the heart increases very little. Alternatively, if the mean arterial pressure (and thus the ventricular pressure) is increased, the oxygen consumption per beat goes up proportionately. In other words, "pressure work" by the heart is far more expensive in terms of O_2 consumption than is "volume work."

A useful index of the cardiac O_2 consumption is the product of mean arterial pressure (more easily measured than the mean ventricular pressure) and the heart rate *(double product)*. Since the duration of systole (and therefore the length of time that the left ventricle must "hold" the mean arterial pressure) does not generally change, this index is usually valid. The heart rate gives the number of times per minute that this pressure must be held. A slightly more accurate prediction of O_2 consumption can be obtained by multiplying heart rate times mean systolic aortic pressure.

These calculations do not take into account the dependence of ventricular pressure development on the radius of the ventricle. The LaPlace relationship states that the heart must develop more tension (force) to generate the same pressure as the radius increases. The extra energy required by pathologically dilated hearts is not reflected in either of the estimates of O_2 consumption outlined above.

Suggested Readings

Berne RM, Levy MN (eds.): *Cardiovascular Physiology.* 4th ed. St. Louis, The C.V. Mosby Company, 1981, pp 71-93

Braunwald E, Ross J: Control of cardiac performance. In *Handbook of Physiology. Section 2. The Cardiovascular System.* Edited by RM Berne, N Sperelakis, SR Geiger. Bethesda, American Physiological Society, 1979, vol. 1, pp 533-580

Hamilton WF, Richards DW: The output of the heart. In *Circulation of the Blood: Men and Ideas.* Edited by AP Fishman and DW Richards. Bethesda, American Physiological Society, 1982, pp 71-126

Katz AM: *Physiology of the Heart.* New York, Raven Press, 1977, chapters 1-13

Murphy RA: Muscle. In *Physiology.* Edited by RM Berne and MN Levy. St. Louis, The C. V. Mosby Company, 1983, 359-406

Chapter 4

Systemic Circulation

This chapter explores the physical principles relating volume, pressure, and the flow of blood in the systemic circulation. In addition, the determinants of the major systemic hemodynamic variables (such as arterial pressure, total peripheral resistance, and blood volume) will be addressed. These general principles form the basis for understanding the regulation of arterial pressure and blood flow to individual tissues, as will be discussed in subsequent chapters.

PRESSURE-FLOW RELATIONSHIP

Fluid flows through a rigid tube only when a pressure (P) gradient exists along its length; the volume flowing per unit time (F) is pro-

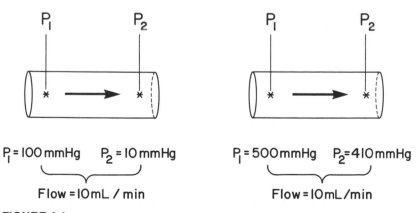

FIGURE 4-1.
Relationship between pressure and flow. Flow is proportional to the pressure *difference* between two points.

portional to the pressure difference between the ends of the tube (fig. 4-1):

$$F = K(P_1 - P_2) = K \times \Delta P$$

$$K = \text{proportionality constant}$$

Let us assume that the pressure difference, ΔP, along the rigid tube in fig. 4-1 is $100 - 10$, or 90 mmHg, and that this produces a flow of 10 mL/min. If the pressure at each end of the tube is raised by 400 mmHg to 500 mmHg and 410 mmHg, respectively, ΔP will still be 90 mmHg, and the flow will remain 10 mL/min. This illustrates that the pressure difference, not the absolute pressure, determines the flow.

Pressure is the force exerted by a fluid on a unit area. In the case of a static fluid, the pressure is the same at any depth regardless of the shape of the container. The pressure at any point in a static column of fluid is therefore proportional to the height of the fluid above that point, and this height is often used as a measure of pressure. The height of a column of mercury is frequently used for this purpose because it is dense (approximately 13 times more dense than water), and a relatively small column height can be employed to measure physiologic pressures (fig. 4-2). For example, mean arterial pressure supports a column of mercury approximately 93 mm high (abbreviated 93 mmHg). If the same arterial pressure were measured by using a column of water, the column would be approximately 4 ft high.[1] Two conventions are observed when measuring blood pressure. First, ambient atmospheric pressure is used as zero reference, so that the mean arterial pressure (mentioned above) is actually 93 mmHg above atmospheric pressure. Second, all cardiovascular pressures are measured at the level of the heart because pressure gradients may vary depending upon position. For example, arterial pressure in the leg of a standing subject is higher than that measured in the arm held at the same level as the heart.

Flow is determined not only by the pressure difference, but also by the value of the proportionality constant, K. The reciprocal of K is the *resistance to flow (R)*, that is, $1/K = R$. In the example in fig. 4-1, R is calculated from the observed values of ΔP and F:

$$F = K \times \Delta P = \frac{\Delta P}{R}$$

and

$$R = \Delta P/F = 90 \text{ mmHg}/10 \text{ mL/min} = 9 \text{ mmHg} \times \text{min/mL} = 9 \text{ PRU}.$$

---

[1]In 1733 Stephen Hales first measured arterial blood pressure by tying a mare to a field gate and placing a long brass tube (which had at its top a glass section) in an artery. The pressure went as high as 8 ft., 3 in. (185 mmHg). The Reverend Mr. Hales pointed out that the heart rate was elevated. You may be reminded of this when you read about the defense response in chapter 5.

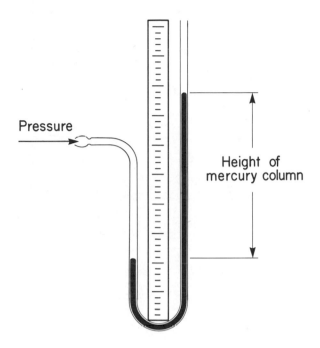

FIGURE 4-2.
Hydrostatic blood pressure. Blood pressure is the height of a column of mercury.

PRU (peripheral resistance unit) is frequently used in place of mmHg × min/mL. Note that resistance is not measured directly, but is calculated from pressure and flow. When fluid flows through a tube, the resistance to flow *(R)* is determined by the properties of both the fluid and the tube. In the case of a steady, streamlined flow of Newtonian fluid through a rigid tube, *Poiseuille's Law*[2] defines the relationship between pressure and flow:

$$F = \Delta P \pi r^4 / 8 \eta L$$

---

[2]Jean Leonard Marie Poiseuille was the first to use mercury for the measurement of blood pressure (1828). After measuring pressures along the aorta and large arteries (where he found little or no pressure drop), he sought to determine the pressures in the small arteries that he could not cannulate. He turned to studies of fluid flow in small tubes, and in doing so developed the basic principles of both hemodynamics and hydrodynamics.

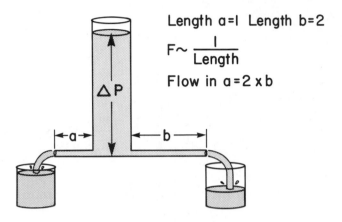

Length a=1 Length b=2

$$F \sim \frac{1}{\text{Length}}$$

Flow in a = 2 x b

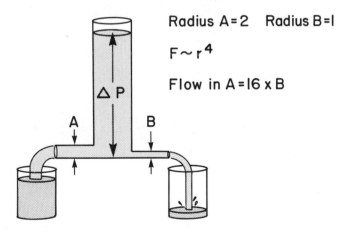

Radius A = 2   Radius B = 1

$$F \sim r^4$$

Flow in A = 16 x B

FIGURE 4-3.
Effect of length and radius of tube on flow.

where r is the radius of the tube, L its length, and η the viscosity of the fluid. Eight and π are geometrical constants. By substitution, the factors determining resistance can be determined:

$$R = 8\,\eta\,L/\,\pi\,r^4.$$

This equation shows that the resistance to blood flow increases proportionately with increases in (1) fluid viscosity or (2) tube length. In contrast, radius changes have a much greater influence because resistance is inversely proportional to the *fourth* power of the radius (see fig. 4-3).

If the conditions indicated in the previous paragraph are not met, Poiseuille's law will not apply. There are several reasons why the cardiovascular system does not strictly meet the criteria necessary to apply Poiseuille's law. First, the cardiovascular system is made up of tapering, branching elastic tubes rather than rigid tubes. Second, blood is not a strict Newtonian fluid. A *Newtonian fluid* is one that exhibits a constant viscosity (η) regardless of flow velocity. When measured *in vitro,* the viscosity of blood decreases as the flow rate increases. This is explained by the observation that red cells tend to collect in the center of the lumen of the vessel as flow velocity increases (fig. 4-4), and this arrangement *(axial streaming)* offers less resistance to flow. This is only a minor effect in the

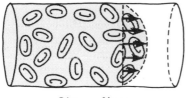
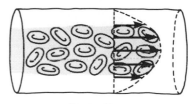

Slow flow   Fast flow

FIGURE 4-4.
Streamline blood flow. As streamline flow velocity increases, the red blood cells collect in the center of the blood vessel and apparent viscosity falls.

range of flow velocities encountered in the body, and we can assume that the viscosity of blood (which is 3 to 4 times that of water) is independent of velocity. However, blood viscosity does increase with hematocrit, as will be discussed below.

Application of Poiseuille's law also requires that flow be stream-lined. *Streamlined (laminar) flow* describes the movement of fluid through a tube in concentric layers that slip past each other. The layers at the center have the fastest velocity, and the layers at the edge of the tube are the slowest. *Turbulent flow* occurs when the following ratio exceeds a critical value called *Reynolds number (Re)*:

$$Re = Vd\rho/\eta$$

where V is the mean velocity, d the tube diameter, ρ the fluid density, and η the fluid viscosity. High flow rates are associated with turbulence. As the pressure gradient along a tube increases, flow and flow velocity increase until the streamlined flow breaks up into eddies and cross-currents, that is, turbulent flow (fig. 4-5). Under

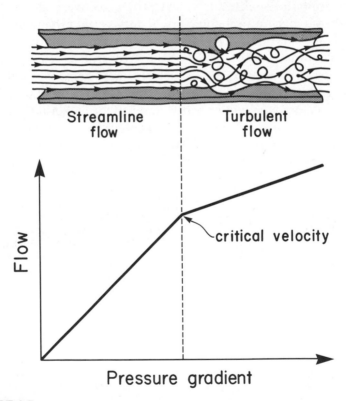

FIGURE 4-5.
Turbulent blood flow. Flow is proportional to the pressure gradient until a critical velocity is reached and turbulent flow results. Because energy is lost in the turbulence, flow does not increase as much for a given rise in pressure after the critical velocity is exceeded. The critical velocity is defined by Reynolds number.

normal circumstances turbulent flow is found only in the aorta, just beyond the aortic valve. Pathologic changes in the cardiac valves or narrowing of arteries can also induce turbulent flow. Turbulent flow results in vibrations that are transmitted to the surface of the body; these vibrations *(bruits and murmurs)* can be heard with a stethoscope.

Although several of the criteria necessary for the strict application of Poiseuille's law are not met, it is extremely useful in thinking about the cardiovascular system. It is widely used as a basis for discussions of the relationship between pressure and flow.

MEAN ARTERIAL PRESSURE

The left ventricle ejects approximately 80 mL of blood into the aorta at a resting rate of 72 times per minute. Pressure subsequently develops in the aorta and large arteries because the distal vasculature imposes a resistance to blood flow from the aorta. Since very little drop in pressure occurs along the aorta and large arteries, the term *arterial pressure* refers to the pressure measured either in the aorta or in any of its major arterial branches. For example, human blood pressure is usually measured in the brachial artery, a third order branch of the aorta that has a slightly (1-3 mmHg) lower pressure than the aorta itself. The aorta and large arteries are sometimes referred to as *conduit vessels* to emphasize the minimal pressure drop along them.

The pressure developed within the aorta and large arteries is determined by two factors: (1) the volume of blood within these vessels and (2) the compliance of the blood vessels. The volume of blood within these vessels depends upon the balance between inflow of blood from the left ventricle and outflow into the distal vessels. On the average (over many cycles of the heart), the flow of blood out of the aorta and major arteries (and into small arteries) equals the flow into the aorta from the heart. However, changes in aortic and large artery volume may occur when inflow and outflow are temporarily imbalanced. The resulting changes in volume will alter the internal pressure and subsequently influence the volume of the blood vessels, as occurs when a balloon is inflated or deflated. The tendency for a vessel to distend when a volume of blood is introduced is called *compliance (C)* and is defined as the change in volume (ΔV) for a given difference in pressure across the vessel wall (P_w):

$$C = \Delta V/P_w.$$

If the pressure on the outside of an artery is equal to atmospheric pressure (and by convention this is made equal to zero), P_w equals arterial pressure, P_a.

The aorta and large arteries fill with blood until the pressure caused by their distention is sufficient to drive the blood out of them (and into the smaller blood vessels) at a flow rate equal to the inflow

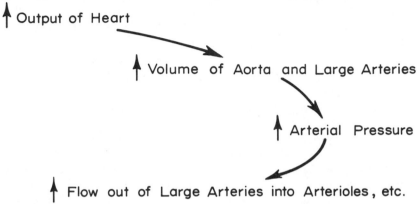

FIGURE 4-6.
Relationship between flow, pressure, and blood vessel volume. The flow of blood from the heart into the aorta is equal to the flow out of the arteries and into the rest of the systemic circulation *only* when the aorta and large arteries are expanded enough to raise arterial pressure to a level that is adequate to push blood on into the small arteries, etc. Whenever a mismatch between flow out of the heart and flow out of the aorta occurs, large vessel volume (and thus arterial pressure) will increase very rapidly and bring the two flows back to equality.

from the heart (fig. 4-6). Flow $(\dot{Q})$ through the aorta and large arteries (equal to the cardiac output in the steady state) is proportional to the pressure difference between the aorta or large arteries (*mean arterial pressure, $\bar{P}_a$*) and the right atrium (right atrial pressure, P_{Ra}):

$$\bar{P}_a - \bar{P}_{Ra} \sim \dot{Q}$$

Since right atrial pressure is normally close to zero and mean arterial pressure is much higher, for example, 93 mmHg, the right atrial pressure is often ignored:

$$\bar{P}_a \sim \dot{Q}$$

Mean arterial pressure is also proportional to the *total peripheral resistance (TPR),* and the inclusion of this term completes the equation:

$$\bar{P}_a = \dot{Q} \times TPR$$

This relationship states that whenever the cardiac output or total peripheral resistance increases, the mean arterial pressure must increase proportionately.

Total peripheral resistance can be calculated from cardiac output and mean arterial pressure because both of these variables can be measured. Bear in mind that cardiac output and total peripheral resistance are the variables that are actually regulated physiologically, and that control of mean arterial pressure is accomplished by adjusting both cardiac output and total peripheral resistance.[3]

PULSE PRESSURE

The pressure in the aorta and large arteries is cyclical, reflecting the cyclical output of the heart; pressure rises with each ejection of blood during left ventricular systole and falls during ventricular diastole. The peak is the *systolic pressure* (P_s); the trough is the *diastolic pressure* (P_d), and the difference between the two pressures is the *pulse pressure*. The mean arterial pressure $(\overline{P}_a)$ is determined mathematically as indicated in fig. 4-7 and is approximately one-third of the pulse pressure added to the diastolic pressure:

$$\overline{P}_a = P_d + \frac{(P_s - P_d)}{3}$$

Mean arterial pressure is not halfway between the diastolic and systolic pressures because the duration of diastole is longer than the duration of systole.

The magnitude of the pulse pressure is determined primarily by the aortic compliance and stroke volume.[4] Each ventricular systole causes an increase in arterial pressure that is proportional to the volume of blood ejected and is inversely proportional to the aortic compliance. The greater the stroke volume the greater the pulse pressure, and the lower the aortic compliance the greater the pulse pressure.

---

[3]This excludes the two indirect ways that mean arterial pressure can affect cardiac output and total peripheral resistance. As indicated in chapter 3, increased mean arterial pressure has the tendency to decrease stroke volume and therefore cardiac output. Increased mean arterial pressure can also stretch arteries and arterioles slightly, thereby lowering total peripheral resistance. The fact remains that the two physiologically controlled variables are cardiac output and total peripheral resistance, and the control of mean arterial pressure depends upon changing these two variables.

[4]Pressure waves reflected from small vessels algebraically add to the pressure determined by these two factors. Because of reflected waves, femoral artery systolic pressure is actually greater than aortic systolic pressure by a few mmHg. Diastolic and mean pressure are lower by 1-2 mmHg in the femoral artery.

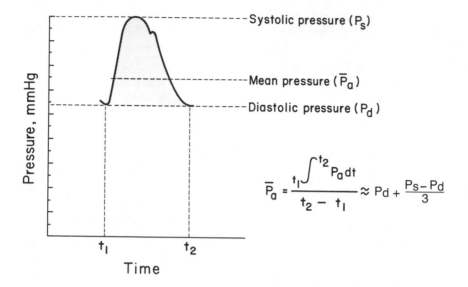

$$\overline{P}_a = \frac{\int_{t_1}^{t_2} P_a\,dt}{t_2 - t_1} \approx P_d + \frac{P_s - P_d}{3}$$

FIGURE 4-7.
Definition of mean arterial pressure. Mean pressure is the area under the pressure curve divided by the time interval, but this can be approximated as one-third the pulse pressure plus the diastolic pressure.

Before considering the effects of various physiologic events upon arterial pressure, one more factor concerning arterial compliance must be introduced. The compliance was previously defined as:

$$C = \Delta V/\Delta P \text{ or } \Delta V = C \times \Delta P$$

Compliance is therefore the slope of the line relating changes in vessel volume to changes in vessel pressure, and it is constant only if the relationship between volume and pressure is linear, as depicted in the left panel of fig. 4-8. In reality, as volume increases the pressure increases disproportionately because the vessel becomes progressively stiffer; that is, compliance decreases with increasing volume. This occurs because the connective tissue sheath *(adventitia)* covering the aorta and large arteries is brought into play as these vessels are stretched. The adventitia resists further stretching (which reduces compliance); therefore, as the mean volume of blood in the aorta increases, a given stroke volume produces a larger pulse pressure.

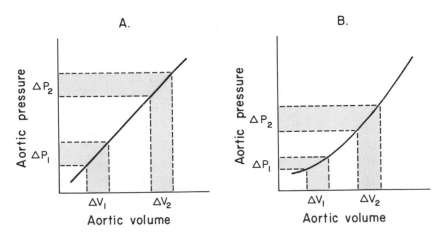

FIGURE 4-8.
Aortic compliance. (A) If the aortic wall were to exhibit linear compliance, a given increase in its volume ($\Delta V_1 = \Delta V_2$) would always result in the same increase in pressure ($\Delta P_1 = \Delta P_2$) regardless of the starting volume. The real case is shown in B. The compliance of the wall decreases as the aorta is inflated. For this reason, the same increase in volume (ΔV_1 or ΔV_2) starting at a higher initial volume results in a greater increase in pressure ($\Delta P_2 > \Delta P_1$).

NORMAL RANGE OF ARTERIAL PRESSURE

The representative numbers usually given for systolic and diastolic pressures are 120 and 80 mmHg, respectively. As is the case for all physiologic variables, values for individuals are distributed around a mean value. For example, in one study of males between the ages of 40 and 45 years, systolic blood pressure averaged 125 mmHg, and 80% of the values fell between 100 and 150 mmHg. Actuarial data generated by various life insurance companies suggest that the normal upper limits for blood pressure (men under 45 years of age) are 140 and 90 mmHg for systolic and diastolic blood pressures, respectively. Increases in mortality have been statistically associated with blood pressures greater than these. However, when blood pressure is assessed, the age of the patient is important because systolic, diastolic, and pulse pressures normally increase with age. Sex, race, and individual habits (such as smoking, certain medications, and a multitude of other factors) can also influence the "normal" blood pressure range.[5] Furthermore, because many variables can transiently

---

[5]Because of this variability, the World Health Organization (WHO) sets a higher arbitrary limit (160/95) on the upper limit of normal for blood pressure than do insurance companies.

affect the blood pressure, several determinations (over time and under various conditions) may be required to make an accurate assessment.

DETERMINANTS OF BLOOD PRESSURE

When total peripheral resistance increases, flow out of the larger arteries is decreased. If cardiac output is unchanged the volume in the aorta and large arteries will increase, as will the mean arterial pressure (fig. 4-9). Mean arterial pressure increases until it is once more

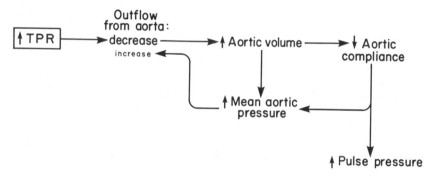

FIGURE 4-9.
Effect of increased TPR on mean arterial and pulse pressure.

sufficient to drive the blood out of the large vessels and into the smaller vessels. At higher aortic volume (and mean arterial pressure), aortic compliance is lower and pulse pressure therefore greater for a given stroke volume (fig. 4-8). The net result is an increase in mean arterial, systolic, and diastolic pressures; the extent to which the pulse pressure increases depends upon how much the arterial compliance decreases with the rise in mean arterial pressure and aortic volume. With older individuals, the fall in compliance for a given increase in mean arterial pressure is greater than it is with younger individuals (fig. 4-10). This explains the higher pulse and systolic pressures that are often observed in older individuals with modest elevations in total peripheral resistance.

Mean arterial pressure is determined only by cardiac output and TPR. For example, an increase in heart rate does not change the mean arterial pressure if the cardiac output remains constant. The

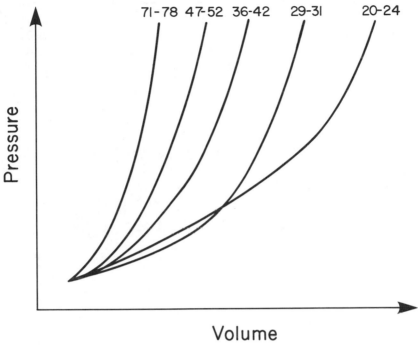

FIGURE 4-10.
Effect of aging on vascular compliance. Relationship between pressure and volume for aortas of humans in different age groups is indicated on curves.

decrease in stroke volume that occurs in this situation results in a diminished pulse pressure; the diastolic pressure increases while the systolic pressure decreases around an unchanged mean arterial pressure (fig. 4-11). An increase in stroke volume with no change in cardiac output likewise causes no change in mean arterial pressure. The increased stroke volume produces a rise in pulse pressure; systolic pressure increases and diastolic pressure decreases.

Another way to think about these events is depicted in fig. 4-12. The first two pressure waves have a diastolic pressure of 80 mmHg, a systolic pressure of 120 mmHg, and a mean arterial pressure of 93 mmHg. The heart rate is 72 beats per minute. After the second beat the heart rate is slowed to 60 beats per minute, but the stroke volume is increased sufficiently to result in the same cardiac output. The longer time interval between beats allows the diastolic pressure to fall to a new (lower) value of 70 mmHg. The next systole, however, produces an increase in the pulse pressure because of the ejection of a greater stroke volume, and the systolic pressure rises to 130

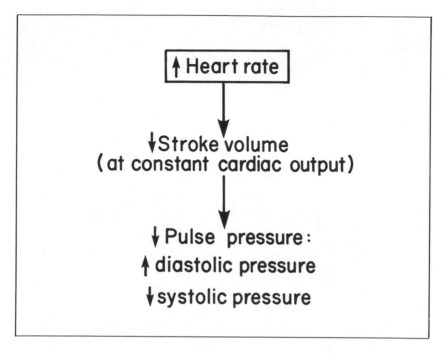

FIGURE 4-11.
Effect of increased heart rate on pulse pressure at constant cardiac output. Mean arterial pressure does not change since cardiac output and total peripheral resistance do not change. Pulse pressure decreases because stroke volume is less.

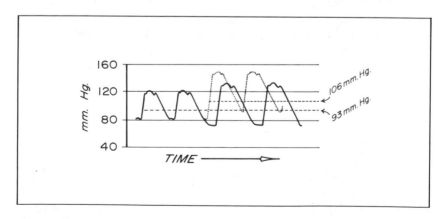

FIGURE 4-12.
Effect of increased stroke volume on arterial pressure with constant (solid lines) and elevated (dotted lines) cardiac output. Total peripheral resistance remains constant.

mmHg. The pressure then falls to the new (lower) diastolic pressure and the cycle is repeated. Mean arterial pressure does not change because the increased pulse pressure is distributed evenly around the same mean. The dashed line shows what would have happened if stroke volume had increased with no change in heart rate. In this case the increased stroke volume would have occurred at the time of the next expected beat, and the diastolic pressure would have been, as for previous beats, 80 mmHg. The increased stroke volume would have resulted in an elevation in systolic pressure to 140 mmHg, after which the pressure would have fallen to a new (higher) diastolic pressure. In this steady state, systolic, diastolic, and mean arterial pressure would all be higher.

Another example is dynamic exercise, for example, running or swimming, which causes an increase in heart rate and stroke volume and a decrease in TPR. Dynamic exercise produces little change in mean arterial pressure because the increase in cardiac output is balanced by the decrease in TPR. Pulse pressure increases due to the increased stroke volume; this results in a relatively lower diastolic and higher systolic pressure (fig. 4-13). These examples demonstrate that mean, systolic, and diastolic pressure can change independent of each other, and that these changes can be predicted from heart rate, stroke volume, and total peripheral resistance.

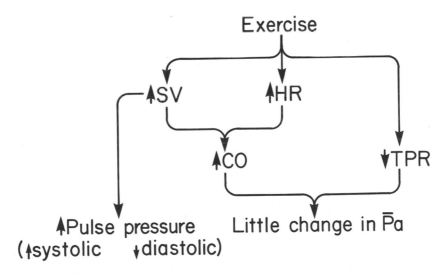

FIGURE 4-13.
Effect of dynamic exercise on mean arterial pressure ($\bar{P}_a$) and pulse pressure.

MEASUREMENT OF ARTERIAL PRESSURE

Arterial blood pressure can be measured by direct or indirect methods. During special testing in hospital settings it is possible to place a catheter in an artery and measure the pressure using electronic transducers. The routine method for measuring human blood pressure is by an indirect procedure using a *sphygmomanometer.* This instrument uses an inflatable cuff that is wrapped around the arm of the patient (fig. 4-14). The cuff is inflated so that the pressure in it

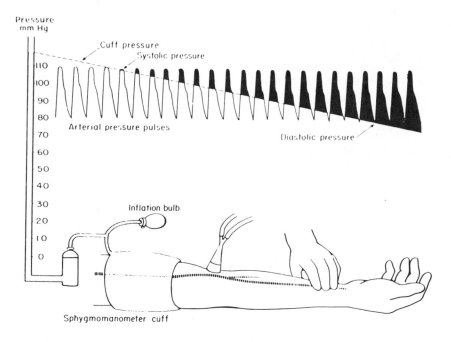

FIGURE 4-14.
Relationship between true arterial pressure and blood pressure as measured with a sphygmomanometer. Reproduced by permission, Rushmer, R.F.: *Cardiovascular Dynamics,* 2nd ed., Philadelphia: W.B. Saunders, 1961, page 155.

exceeds the systolic pressure of the subject. The external pressure compresses the arteries and cuts off blood flow into the limb. The air in the cuff is then slowly released, and a stethoscope placed over the brachial artery distal to it is used to determine when the noise due to the turbulent flow of blood pushing under the cuff *(Korotkoff sound)* is first heard. The pressure corresponding to this first appearance of blood pushing under the cuff is the systolic pressure. The turbulent flow of blood under the cuff results from the pinching of the brachial artery and the resulting high flow velocity. As pressure in the cuff continues to fall, the brachial artery resumes its normal shape and both the abnormal turbulence and the noise cease. The pressure at which the noise ceases is taken to be the diastolic pressure. This is obviously a simplified explanation of the physiology involved, and the accurate determination of blood pressure by this method is influenced by an assortment of variables. For example, in the elderly (or in those with "stiff" or hard-to-compress blood vessels from other causes, such as diabetes) additional external pressure may be required to compress the blood vessels and stop flow. This extra pressure gives a falsely high estimate of the blood pressure. Obesity may likewise contribute to an inaccurate assessment.

TOTAL PERIPHERAL RESISTANCE

Total peripheral resistance (TPR) is the frictional resistance to blood flow provided by all of the vessels between the large arteries and right atrium, including the small arteries, arterioles, capillaries, venules, small veins, and veins. The relative importance of the various segments contributing to the total peripheral resistance can be appreciated by observing the profile of the pressure drop along the vascular tree (fig. 4-15). Note that very little change in pressure occurs in the aorta and large arteries. Approximately 70% of the pressure drop occurs in the small arteries and arterioles, and another 20% of the drop occurs in the capillaries. The small arteries and arterioles are the primary regulators of total peripheral resistance. Contraction and relaxation of the smooth muscle in their walls changes their radius, which in turn influences the flow of blood through them.

To emphasize the importance of smooth muscle in the control of TPR, consider the role of each factor in Poiseuille's law:

$$R = 8\eta \, L/\pi \, r^4$$

The potential influences on resistance are blood viscosity, vessel length, and radius. Viscosity increases with hematocrit (fig. 4-16),

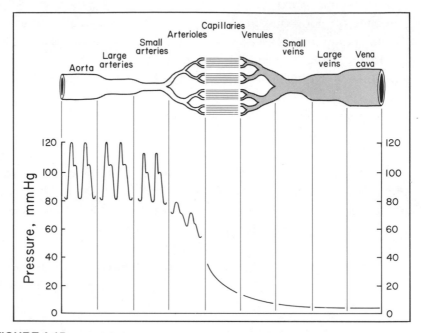

FIGURE 4-15.
Pressure in different vessels of the systemic circulation.

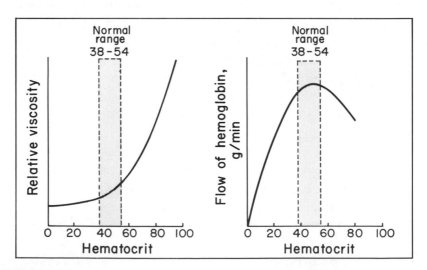

FIGURE 4-16.
Effect of hematocrit on blood viscosity. Because of the sharp increase in viscosity produced by above-normal hematocrits (causing an increase in resistance to flow), little increase in the delivery of hemoglobin and oxygen occurs when the hematocrit rises above the normal range.

especially when the hematocrit is above the normal range of 38% - 54%. As a result of the increase in viscosity, the oxygen-carrying capacity provided by the greater number of red blood cells is offset by the increase in resistance to flow. Individuals with *polycythemia* (increased mass or number of red blood cells) may actually deliver less oxygen to tissues during exercise because of increased viscosity, despite the enhanced oxygen-carrying capacity provided by the extra red blood cells. The normal hematocrit reflects the correct balance between sufficient red blood cells for oxygen carriage and the negative effect of additional red blood cells on the resistance to blood flow.

Despite the potential effect of blood viscosity on resistance, hematocrit does not change very much under most physiological conditions and is usually not an important determinant of vascular resistance. The length of blood vessels likewise does not change significantly and is therefore not important as a physiologic determinant of vascular resistance. The remaining influence, vessel radius, is

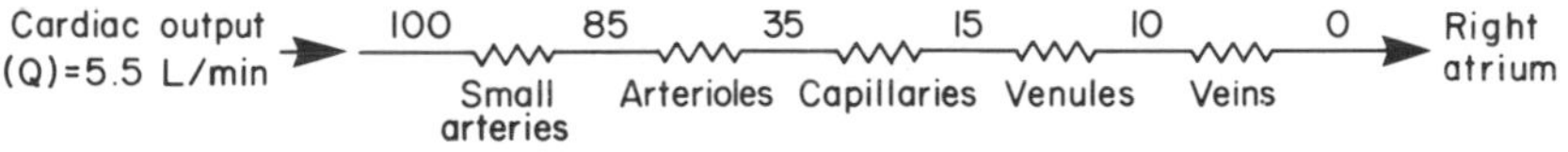

$$\frac{\Delta P}{Q} = R$$

Resistances

Small arteries	$\frac{100-85}{5.5}$	= 2.73
Arterioles	$\frac{85-35}{5.5}$	= 9.09
Capillaries	$\frac{35-15}{5.5}$	= 3.64
Venules	$\frac{15-10}{5.5}$	= 0.91
Veins	$\frac{10-0}{5.5}$	= 1.82

Total = 18.18

Total peripheral resistance (TPR) = $\frac{100-0}{5.5}$ = 18.18

FIGURE 4-17.
Resistances in series. Resistances in series are added to obtain the total resistance. In this case the resistances of consecutive vascular segments are added to obtain the total peripheral resistance. The quantity ΔP is the difference in pressure across the resistance. Q = cardiac output.

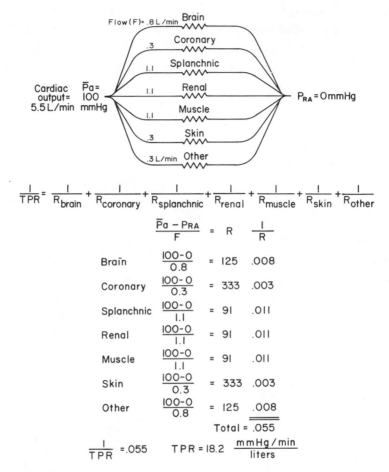

$$\frac{1}{TPR} = \frac{1}{R_{brain}} + \frac{1}{R_{coronary}} + \frac{1}{R_{splanchnic}} + \frac{1}{R_{renal}} + \frac{1}{R_{muscle}} + \frac{1}{R_{skin}} + \frac{1}{R_{other}}$$

	$\dfrac{\bar{P}a - P_{RA}}{F}$	= R	$\dfrac{1}{R}$
Brain	$\dfrac{100-0}{0.8}$	= 125	.008
Coronary	$\dfrac{100-0}{0.3}$	= 333	.003
Splanchnic	$\dfrac{100-0}{1.1}$	= 91	.011
Renal	$\dfrac{100-0}{1.1}$	= 91	.011
Muscle	$\dfrac{100-0}{1.1}$	= 91	.011
Skin	$\dfrac{100-0}{0.3}$	= 333	.003
Other	$\dfrac{100-0}{0.8}$	= 125	.008

Total = .055

$$\frac{1}{TPR} = .055 \qquad TPR = 18.2 \ \frac{mmHg/min}{liters}$$

FIGURE 4-18.
Resistances in parallel. The resistance of the parallel organ circuits cannot be added directly to obtain TPR. Instead, the reciprocals of each organ resistance must be added to obtain the reciprocal of TPR. $\bar{P}_a$ = mean arterial pressure, P_{RA} = right atrial pressure.

therefore the major determinant of changes in the total peripheral resistance. Since resistance is proportional to r^4, small changes in the radius cause relatively large changes in vascular resistance. For example, during exercise the vascular resistance of skeletal muscle may decrease by 25-fold. This fall in resistance results from a 2.2-fold increase in the resistance vessel radius, that is, $2.2^4 \approx 25$. The vessel radius is primarily determined by the contractile activity of the smooth muscle in the vessel wall, and the control of vascular smooth muscle will be considered in detail in chapter 6.

TPR is the net result of resistance offered by many vessels arranged both in series and in parallel, and it is worth considering the effects of vessel arrangement on total resistance. Resistances in series are simply summed;[6] for example:

$$TPR = R_{small\ arteries} + R_{arterioles} +$$
$$R_{capillaries} + R_{venules} + R_{small\ veins}$$

(fig. 4-17). For resistance in parallel, it is the reciprocal of the parallel resistances that are summed (fig. 4-18).

BLOOD VOLUME

The blood volume is distributed among the various portions of the circulatory system according to the pattern shown in fig. 4-19. Approximately 80% is located in the *systemic circulation,* [7] and 60% (or 75% of the systemic blood volume) is located on the venous

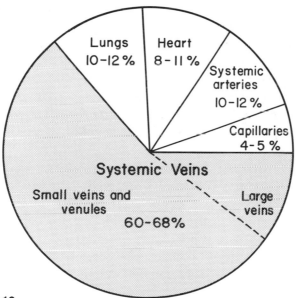

FIGURE 4-19.
Blood volumes of various elements of the circulation in the resting individual.

---

[6]Those who remember their physics may have noted already that pressure difference is analogous to potential (as is blood flow to current); the ratio of potential to current is electrical resistance. Resistances in series and in parallel are treated the same way in the analysis of electrical and hydraulic circuits.

[7]The systemic blood volume is the total volume minus the volume in the heart and lungs.

side of the circulation. The volume of blood present in the arteries and capillaries is only 20% of the total blood volume. Since most of the systemic blood volume is in veins, it is not surprising that changes in systemic blood volume primarily reflect changes in venous volume.

Veins are approximately 20 times more compliant than arteries; small changes in venous pressure are therefore associated with large changes in venous volume. If 1000 mL of blood is infused into the circulation, 95% (or 950 mL) ends up in veins and only 5% (50 mL) in arteries.

In considering the venous side of the circulation, it is useful to divide the blood volume into an intrathoracic *(central)* blood volume and an extrathoracic peripheral blood volume. The central blood volume includes the blood in the superior and intrathoracic portions of the inferior vena cava, right atrium and ventricle, pulmonary circulation, and left atrium; this constitutes approximately 50% of the total blood volume. From a functional standpoint, the most important components of the extrathoracic blood volume are those volumes of blood in the extremities and abdominal cavity. The blood in the neck and head is less important because (1) there is far less blood in these regions, and (2) the blood volume inside the cranium cannot change because the skull is rigid. In contrast, the veins of the extremities and abdominal cavity are of considerable functional importance because large changes in their blood volume can occur.

Cardiac output is extremely sensitive to the effects of central blood volume on left ventricular end diastolic fiber length (see chapter 3). For example, if blood is infused into the inferior vena cava of a normal subject, the volume of blood returning to the chest (venous return) will be transiently greater than the volume leaving it (the cardiac output). This difference between the input and output of blood produces an increase in the right atrial pressure, which in turn increases right ventricular end diastolic fiber length and therefore right heart stroke volume. Flow through the lungs to the left heart will subsequently rise and cause a proportional increase in left heart stroke volume. This process will raise cardiac output until it equals the sum of the venous return to the heart (by way of the inferior and superior vena cavae) plus the infused blood. The central blood volume is therefore a critical determinant of the cardiac output.

Two important factors influence the central blood volume: (1) changes in total blood volume and (2) changes in the distribution of fixed blood volumes between intrathoracic and extrathoracic regions. An increase in total blood volume can occur because of an infusion of fluid, retention of salt and water by the kidneys, or a shift in fluid from the interstitial space to plasma. A decrease in blood volume can occur because of hemorrhage, losses through sweat or other body fluids, or the transfer of fluid from plasma into the interstitial space. Changes in blood volume that are unaccompanied by shifts in distribution result in proportional changes in both central blood volume and extrathoracic blood volume. For example, a moderate hemorrhage (10% of blood volume) with no distribution shift would cause a 10% decrease in central blood volume. The reduced intrathoracic blood volume would, in the absence of compensatory events, lead to decreased filling of the ventricles with diminished stroke volume and cardiac output.

Shifts in the distribution of blood volume occur because of (1) changes in the transmural pressures of the vessels and/or (2) changes in the compliance of either the extrathoracic or the intrathoracic vessels. The best example of a change in transmural pressure occurs whenever an individual stands up. Standing increases the pressure in the blood vessels of the legs because it creates a column of blood between the heart and leg blood vessels. The arterial and venous pressures of the ankles during standing can easily be 130 cm (4.3 ft) of water (blood), which is 100 mmHg higher than in the recumbent position. The increased transmural pressure (outside pressure is still atmospheric) results in little distention of arteries because of their low compliance, but in considerable distention of veins because of their high compliance. In fact, approximately 550 mL of blood is needed to fill the stretched veins of the legs and feet when an average person stands up.[8] The blood is obtained from the central blood volume by the following sequence of events (fig. 4-20). When a person stands, blood continues to be pumped by the heart at the same rate and stroke volume for one or two beats. However, much of the blood reaching the legs remains in the veins as they become passively stretched to their new size by the increased venous (transmural) pressure. This, in turn, decreases the return of blood to the chest. Since cardiac output exceeds venous

---

[8]It is interesting to note that standing would have no effect upon flow if arteries and veins were rigid tubes. As in the case of a siphon, whatever pressures were added to the venous side of the circulation would also be added to the arterial side; thus the increased pressures would exactly balance. See chapter 8.

return for a few beats, the central blood volume falls (as does the end diastolic fiber length, stroke volume, and cardiac output). Once the veins of the legs reach their new steady state volume, the venous return again equals cardiac output. The equality between venous return and cardiac output occurs even though the central blood volume is now reduced by 550 mL. The new cardiac output and venous return are decreased because of the reduction in central blood volume.

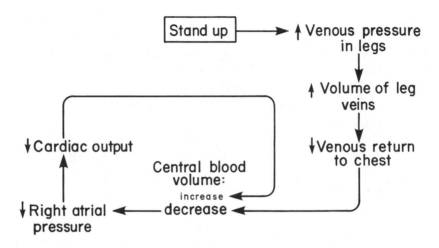

FIGURE 4-20.
Effect of standing on central blood volume and cardiac output.

Compensatory mechanisms minimize the effects of the above events and will be discussed in detail in chapter 8. One of these compensatory events illustrates the other way in which the distribution of blood volume can be altered, which is by a change in venous compliance. If the smooth muscle in the walls of leg veins contracts when a person stands, this decreases the compliance of these veins. Less volume is needed to fill the veins because of the lower compliance, and less shift from the central blood volume to the extrathoracic blood volume occurs.

Clinicians and physiologists have tried to use venous pressure measurements to monitor the types of events discussed above. Unfortunately, measurements of the peripheral venous pressure, such as the pressure in an arm or leg vein, are subject to too many influences (such as partial occlusion caused by positioning) to be very helpful in most clinical situations. Central venous pressure can be measured by placing a catheter in the superior vena cava, inferior vena cava, or right atrium via a large vein. It is often a good indicator of central blood volume because the compliance of the intrathoracic vessels usually does not change much. In certain situations, however, such as with tricuspid valve insufficiency, the physiologic meaning of central venous pressure is changed because right ventricular pressure is transmitted to the right atrium during ventricular systole. The use of central venous pressure as an estimate of central blood volume depends upon the assumption that the right heart is pumping normally.

In summary, it should be appreciated that (1) volume shifts could not occur without the high compliance of veins; (2) volume shifts involve changes in central blood volume, which in turn affect stroke volume and cardiac output; and (3) changes in central blood volume are the result of transient imbalances between cardiac output and venous return. These principles will be used in later chapters to explain the overall performance of the cardiovascular system.

Suggested Readings

Berne RM, Levy MN (eds.): *Cardiovascular Physiology.* 4th ed. St. Louis, The C. V. Mosby Company, 1981, pp 52-70, 94-108

Cokelet GR: Hemodynamics. In *Peripheral Circulation.* Edited by PC Johnson. New York, John Wiley and Sons, 1978, pp 81-110

Pickering G: Systemic arterial hypertension. In *Circulation of the Blood: Men and Ideas.* Edited by AP Fishman and DW Richards. Bethesda, American Physiological Society, 1982, pp 3-70

Chapter 5

Neural and Hormonal Control of the Circulation

Central blood volume and arterial pressure are regulated by a number of neural and hormonal mechanisms. Neural control involves both sympathetic and parasympathetic branches of the autonomic nervous system. Blood volume and arterial pressure are monitored by stretch receptors in the heart and arteries. Afferent nerve traffic from these receptors is integrated in the brain stem, which leads to levels of activity in sympathetic and parasympathetic nerves that adjust cardiac output and total peripheral resistance to maintain arterial pressure. Sympathetic nerve activity and, even more important, hormones such as vasopressin, renin, angiotensin, aldosterone, and several others serve as effectors for the regulation of salt and water balance and blood volume. Neural control of cardiac output and total peripheral resistance is most important in the minute-to-minute regulation of arterial pressure, whereas hormones are most important in long-term regulation of arterial pressure.

In some situations factors other than blood volume and arterial pressure regulation dominate cardiovascular control mechanisms. These situations include the defense response, certain types of exercise, diving, and thermoregulation.

AUTONOMIC CONTROL

The *parasympathetic* and *sympathetic* divisions of the autonomic nervous system participate in cardiovascular control. The following sections will describe these systems as they relate to the cardiovascular system.

FUNCTIONAL ANATOMY
The autonomic pathways are composed of two neurons that link the

central nervous system (spinal cord or brain) with target organs (fig. 5-1). In the case of the parasympathetic nervous system, the cell

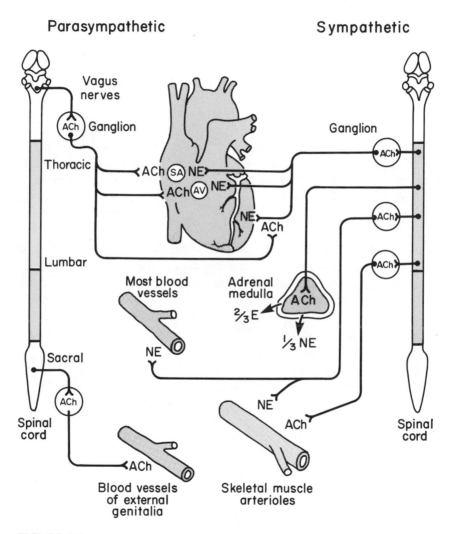

FIGURE 5-1.
Autonomic innervation of the cardiovascular system. ACh = acetylcholine, NE = norepinephrine, E = epinephrine, SA = sinoatrial node, AV = atrio-ventricular node.

body of the first neuron is located in either the brain stem or the sacral segment of the spinal cord (for this reason, the parasympathetic nervous system is often called the *craniosacral*). This first neuron is called a *preganglionic* neuron. The preganglionic neuron synapses with nearby neurons within the spinal cord and with neurons from higher levels in the spinal cord and brain. After leaving the central nervous system, it synapses with the second, or *postganglionic,* neuron in a ganglion located within (or adjacent to) the organ that it supplies. The postganglionic neuron releases its neurotransmitter directly upon cells of the target organ.

The cell bodies of the sympathetic preganglionic neurons are located in the thoracic and lumbar segments of the spinal cord (the sympathetic nervous system is therefore also referred to as the *thoracolumbar* division of the autonomic nervous system). The preganglionic and postganglionic sympathetic fibers synapse in ganglia located along the thoracic and lumbar segments of the spinal cord, and in a few ganglia within the abdominal cavity. Postganglionic fibers then run to most organs, where the neurotransmitter is released upon cells of the target organ.

All parasympathetic preganglionic and postganglionic fibers, as well as all preganglionic sympathetic fibers, release acetylcholine; most sympathetic postganglionic neurons release norepinephrine, but a few neurons ending on skeletal muscle arterioles release acetylcholine.

The one exception to the general scheme of preganglionic and postganglionic fibers outlined above is the innervation of the adrenal medulla. In this tissue, preganglionic sympathetic fibers end directly upon adrenal medullary cells (fig. 5-1). Acetylcholine is the neurotransmitter and causes the adrenal medulla to release a mixture of norepinephrine (one-third) and epinephrine (two-thirds). This exception is not difficult to understand when it is remembered that the adrenal medullary cells have the same embryologic origin as the postganglionic neurons of the sympathetic nervous system.

The heart receives innervation from both the sympathetic and parasympathetic nervous system. This double source of innervation—with opposing effects—is known as *dual innervation,* and it enhances the degree to which autonomic responses can be "finetuned." In general, when the sympathetic nervous output to the heart increases, the parasympathetic nervous output decreases, and vice versa. The ventricles receive relatively sparse innervation from the parasympathetic nervous system. Most parasympathetic fibers probably end upon sympathetic nerves and influence release of norepinephrine (see below). Most blood vessels, with the exception of those of the external genitalia and the heart, receive only sympathetic innervation. Those of the external genitalia and heart also receive parasympathetic innervation.[1]

NEUROTRANSMITTERS

Neurotransmitters released from autonomic neurons include norepinephrine, acetylcholine, and a variety of other substances including dopamine, vasoactive intestinal peptide, and ATP. The physiologic significance of the latter neurotransmitters has not been fully worked out and will not be discussed here. They are mentioned to forewarn the student that the neurochemistry of the cardiovascular system is changing rapidly, and there will be major new pharmacologic approaches to the treatment of cardiovascular disease in the future.

NOREPINEPHRINE

Most postganglionic sympathetic neurons release *norepinephrine.* Norepinephrine is stored in *varicosities* of the sympathetic nerve terminals, which are located very close to cardiac or vascular smooth muscle (fig. 5-2). These varicosities contain vesicles that are spherical lipid membranes containing norepinephrine, dopamine, and dopamine β-hydroxylase. Norepinephrine is synthesized in the varicosities (fig. 5-3). Action potentials reaching the varicosities result in the opening of voltage-dependent Ca^{2+} channels. Increased Ca^{2+} concentration within the varicosity causes some of the vesicles to fuse with the interior of the plasma membrane and release their contents (fig. 5-4). This process is called *exocytosis.*

The number of vesicles that release their products is partially dependent upon the rate at which action potentials reach the varicosity. However, there are a number of potent modifiers of the relationship between action potential frequency and vesicular release of norepinephrine. Several agents inhibit the release of norepinephrine. These include norepinephrine itself, which exerts a negative feedback effect inhibiting further norepinephrine release. Acetylcholine, released from cholinergic nerve endings, also inhibits the release of norepinephrine. Finally, a number of locally re-

---

[1]Despite these two examples, parasympathetic innervation of *blood vessels* plays no significant role in regulation of blood pressure. Contrary to the claims of certain *macho* medical students, activation of these fibers cannot cause hypotension.

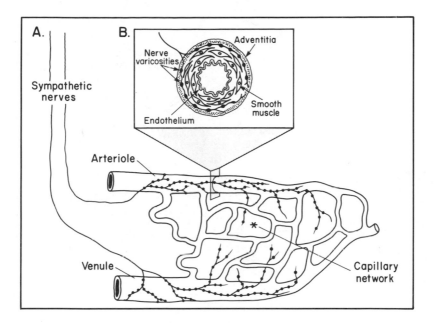

FIGURE 5-2.
Sympathetic innervation of blood vessels. (A) Sympathetic nerve terminals containing varicosities anastamose freely in the adventitia of arteries and veins. The smallest vessels in the microcirculation are not heavily innervated. (B) The varicosities are located in the outer portions of the vascular wall.

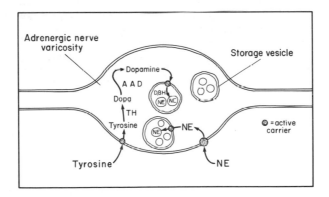

FIGURE 5-3.
Synthesis of norepinephrine. Norepinephrine is synthesized in the adrenergic varicosities from tyrosine. Tyrosine is transported into the varicosity where tyrosine hydroxylase (TH) catalyzes the formation of dopa. The conversion of dopa to dopamine is catalyzed by aromatic-L-amino acid decarboxylase (AAD). Dopamine is transported into the storage vesicle, where it is acted upon by dopamine β-hydroxylase (DβH) to form norepinephrine. Preformed norepinephrine can also enter the varicosities and then the vesicle.

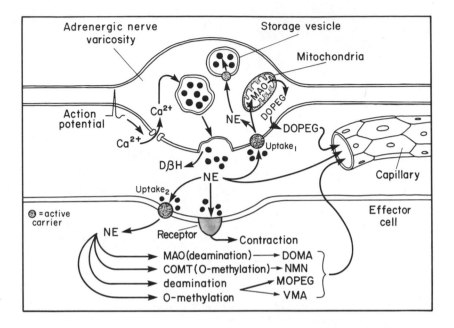

FIGURE 5-4.

Release and metabolism of norepinephrine. Action potentials in sympathetic nerves result in the opening of Ca^{2+} channels in varicosities. Increased Ca^{2+} in the neuron cytosol causes exocytotic release of norepinephrine (NE) from the vesicles. Norepinephrine released into the neuromuscular cleft binds to receptors in the muscle membrane. It is removed by uptake into nerve (uptake 1) or muscle (uptake 2) cells. In nerve cells it is oxidized to 3,4-dehydroxyphenylglycol (DOPEG) by monoamine oxidase (MAO). In muscle cells it undergoes oxidation and/or deamination by MAO and catechol-O-methyl transferase (COMT), respectively. Four products result: 3,4-dihydroxymandelic acid (DOMA); normetanephrine (NMN); 3-methoxy, 4-dihydroxyphenylglycol (MOPEG); and 3-methoxy, 4-hydroxymandelic acid (VMA). These substances join NE and DOPEG in the capillary effluent from the region. Dopamine β-hydroxylase is likewise contained in the vesicles and is released by exocytosis; this enzyme also leaves the tissue via capillary blood flow.

leased substances including prostaglandins, serotonin, ATP, adenosine, and K^+ reduce norepinephrine release. In contrast, angiotensin II enhances norepinephrine release. All of these agents, with the exception of K^+, act on receptor molecules in the plasma membrane of the varicosities. Norepinephrine is removed from the neuromuscular junction by (1) uptake into the nerve varicosities or into the effector cells and (2) by diffusion out of the neurotransmitter junction to nearby capillaries (fig. 5-4).

ADRENERGIC RECEPTORS

Adrenergic receptors are protein molecules contained in the plasma membranes of cardiac muscle, vascular smooth muscle, and nerve varicosities. They are classified according to their ability to bind different *agonists* (i.e., norepinephrine, epinephrine, and a series of chemical analogues) and *antagonists* (drugs that block the action of the agonists). They are *not* classified according to the action they mediate. The student must learn to identify these receptors by their affinities to agonists and antagonists. We will define adrenergic receptors and their subtypes by (1) their ability to bind to the agonists norepinephrine and epinephrine, and to their chemical analogues, phenylephrine and isoproterenol; and (2) their ability to bind several antagonists (table 5-1).

Table 5-1. Binding Affinities of Adrenergic Receptors for Agonists and Antagonists

	Alpha Receptors		Beta Receptors	
	Subtype 1	Subtype 2	Subtype 1	Subtype 2
Agonists				
Norepinephrine	+ + + +	+ + + +	+ + +	+
Epinephrine	+ +	+ +	+ +	+ + + +
Phenylephrine	+ + + +	+	0	0
Isoproterenol	+	+	+ + + +	+ + + +
Antagonists				
Phentolamine	+ + + +	+ + + +	0	0
Prazosin	+ + + +	+	0	0
Propranolol	0	0	+ + + +	+ + + +
Atenolol	0	0	+ + + +	0

NOTE: Adrenergic receptor type and subtypes are defined by their affinity for these and other substances. They are not defined by the action that they mediate.
+ + + + = strongly binds   0 = does not bind

ALPHA-ADRENERGIC RECEPTORS

Alpha-adrenergic receptors (table 5-2) bind norepinephrine and phenylephrine with a higher affinity than they bind epinephrine and isoproterenol. It is useful to subdivide α-receptors into α_1- and α_2-receptors (table 5-1). Alpha$_1$-receptors have a high affinity for the antagonists phentolamine and prazosin, whereas α_2-receptors have a high affinity for phentolamine, but not prazosin. Alpha$_1$-receptors are found in the plasma membranes of vascular smooth muscle cells from arteries and veins of all sizes. When an agonist, for

Table 5-2. Adrenergic Receptors: Location, Action Mediated, and Source of Agonist

Receptor Type	Location	Action	Physiologic Agonist
alpha$_1$	Smooth muscle of arteries and veins	Contraction	Norepinephrine from postganglionic sympathetics
alpha$_2$	Sympathetic nerve varicosities	Inhibition of norepinephrine release	Norepinephrine from postganglionic sympathetics
	Central nervous system	Inhibition of sympathetic neural output	Norepinephrine from central neurons
beta$_1$	Sinoatrial node	Increased heart rate	Norepinephrine from postganglionic sympathetics
	Atrial and ventricular muscle	Increased conduction velocity and contractility	Norepinephrine from postganglionic sympathetics
	Atrioventricular node and Purkinje system	Increased conduction velocity	Norepinephrine from postganglionic sympathetics
beta$_2$	Smooth muscle of arteries and veins	Relaxation	Epinephrine from adrenal medulla

example, norepinephrine, binds to this type of receptor, contraction occurs because of an increase in cytosolic Ca^{2+} concentration.

Alpha$_2$-receptors are found in the plasma membranes of sympathetic varicosities. Norepinephrine binding to these receptors inhibits norepinephrine release from the varicosity. This serves as a negative feedback mechanism to limit the concentration of norepinephrine in the neuroeffector junction. Alpha$_2$-receptors are also found in the central nervous system, where they mediate inhibition of sympathetic output.

BETA-ADRENERGIC RECEPTORS
Beta-adrenergic receptors (table 5-2) have a high affinity for epinephrine and isoproterenol. In addition, they bind the antagonist propranolol. Beta-receptors can be subdivided into β_1- and β_2-receptors (table 5-1). Beta$_1$-receptors have a higher affinity for norepinephrine and the antagonist atenolol than do β_2-receptors. Beta$_1$-receptors are found in the plasma membranes of cardiac cells, where they cause an increased rate of depolarization (in pacemaker cells—see chapter 2), increased velocity of conduction of action

potentials, and increased contractility. All of these effects are initiated by the activation of adenylate cyclase (chapter 3).

Beta$_2$-receptors are found in the plasma membranes of vascular smooth muscle cells. They are most prevalent in the smooth muscle of coronary and skeletal muscle arterioles. The physiologic agonist for these receptors is circulating epinephrine. Epinephrine binding to these receptors activates adenylate cyclase and leads to relaxation of vascular smooth muscle (chapter 6).

ACETYLCHOLINE

Acetylcholine is released from all preganglionic sympathetic and parasympathetic fibers, all postganglionic parasympathetic fibers, and postganglionic sympathetic fibers to arterioles of skeletal muscles. Release of acetylcholine from postganglionic neurons is shown in fig. 5-5. Acetylcholine is formed in nerve endings from choline and acetyl CoA. Choline is actively transported into the nerve endings and acetyl CoA is made by mitochondria located there. Choline acetyltransferase catalyzes the esterification of these two substances to form acetylcholine, which is stored in synaptic vesicles. The arrival of an action potential causes the entry of Ca^{2+}, which leads to release of acetylcholine by exocytosis. Acetylcholine is rapidly broken down by acetylcholine esterase in the neuroeffector junction.

There are two classes of acetylcholine receptors (table 5-3). One class, the *nicotinic receptors,* is found primarily in sympathetic and parasympathetic ganglia. These receptors are located in the plasma membrane of postganglionic neurons and adrenal medullary cells. They have a high affinity for the agonists acetylcholine and nicotine and for the antagonist hexamethonium. The receptor is a transmembrane protein that serves as a cation channel. When it binds to acetylcholine the channel opens, allowing the passage of K^+ and Na^+. This results in depolarization of the membrane.

The other class of acetylcholine receptors, the *muscarinic receptors,* is located in the plasma membranes of cardiac and vascular smooth muscle cells, endothelial cells, and sympathetic varicosities. These receptors have a high affinity for the agonists acetylcholine and muscarine[2] and the antagonist atropine.

Acetylcholine binding to the muscarinic receptor causes slowing of heart rate (see chapter 2), lowered conduction velocity in

---

[2]Muscarine is a toxin found in some toadstools.

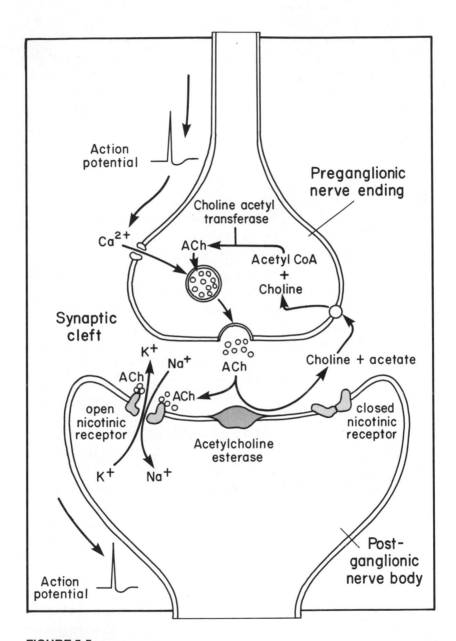

FIGURE 5-5.
Release and metabolism of acetylcholine. Preganglionic cholinergic nerve endings synapse with postganglionic nerves. Acetylcholine (synthesized via choline acetyltransferase) is packaged into synaptic vesicles and released by action potentials. The action potential causes Ca^{2+} channels in the membrane to open; this enables Ca^{2+} to enter, which in turn causes exocytosis.

Table 5-3. Acetylcholine Receptors: Location, Action Mediated, and Source of Agonist

Receptor Type	Location	Action	Physiologic Agonist
Nicotinic	Postganglionic neurons of autonomic nervous system	Excitation of postganglionic neurons	Acetylcholine from preganglionic neurons
Muscarinic	Sinoatrial node	Slowing of heart rate	Acetylcholine from postganglionic parasympathetics
	Atrioventricular node and specialized conducting tissues	Slowing of conduction velocity	Acetylcholine from postganglionic parasympathetics
	Arterioles[a] of skeletal muscle	Vasodilation	Acetylcholine from postganglionic sympathetics
	Arterioles[a] of heart, brain, and external genitalia	Vasodilation	Acetylcholine from postganglionic parasympathetics
	Most other blood vessels[a]	Vasodilation	None known. Acetylcholine does not ordinarily circulate, and there are no cholinergic nerves to these vessels
	Sympathetic varicosities	Inhibition of norepinephrine release	Acetylcholine from postganglionic parasympathetics

[a]In many cases, the muscarinic receptors that mediate vasodilation may be located in the plasma membrane of endothelial cells, not in the vascular smooth muscle cells.

cardiac cells, relaxation of vascular smooth muscle,[3] and inhibition of the release of norepinephrine from sympathetic varicosities. The cellular mechanism of these effects is still being worked out. We know that there are plasma membrane effects that cause the opening of K^+ leak channels and hyperpolarization in cardiac cells. We also know that guanylate cyclase activation is involved and that cyclic GMP may act as a second messenger.

CNS AREAS INVOLVED IN CONTROL OF THE CARDIOVASCULAR SYSTEM

SPINAL

Some spinal reflexes of cardiovascular significance occur in hu-

---

[3]This effect is mediated via endothelial cells as will be discussed in chapter 6.

mans. For example, the stimulation of pain fibers entering the spinal cord below the level of a cord transection can cause reflex vasoconstriction and increased blood pressure. In addition, neural pathways from higher centers may converge at the level of the spinal cord, allowing the final integration of various neural activities to occur.

MEDULLARY

The major area for the integration of the simple reflex behavior of the cardiovascular system is the medulla oblongata. The medullary cardiovascular neurons are grouped in three distinct pools that lead to activation of (1) sympathetic neurons to the blood vessels, (2) sympathetic neurons to the heart, and, (3) parasympathetic neurons to the heart. The first two (1 and 2) are often called the *vasomotor center* and the third (3) the *cardio-inhibitory center.* All three neuron pools interconnect extensively; it is on this level that the push-pull firing of parasympathetic and sympathetic fibers to the heart is actually integrated. Because of this integration, it seems reasonable to call the entire area the *medullary cardiovascular center* and not attempt to distinguish between the various subdivisions.

CORTICAL

The highest levels of organization in the autonomic nervous system are the *corticohypothalamic* pathways that orchestrate various cardiovascular correlates to different patterns of behavior. For example, when certain areas of the hypothalamus of cats are stimulated, a characteristic rage response occurs with spitting, clawing, tail lashing, arched back, etc. An accompanying characteristic set of cardiovascular responses, including tachycardia and elevated blood pressure, also occurs. If certain connections between the hypothalamus and the cerebral cortex are severed, cats will exhibit this rage reaction even when they are not being threatened. The reaction apparently is due to the loss of pathways that normally exert inhibitory influences upon the hypothalamic center. Details of the defense response and other examples of combined corticohypothalamic behavior and cardiovascular events will be described below. The important points here are that multiple connections between the cerebral cortical, hypothalamic, medullary, and spinal levels of the autonomic nervous system exist, and that corticohypothalamic pathways integrate many behavioral and cardiovascular patterns involving such activities as fighting, eating, diving, and thermoregulation.

NEUROTRANSMITTERS IN THE CNS

A very large number of neurotransmitters play a role in the central regulation of cardiovascular function. Their specific roles are just beginning to be understood. Among the better described are (1) norepinephrine, which acts in the medulla via α_2-receptors to inhibit sympathetic neural traffic to the heart and blood vessels (this is the basis by which the central action of the α_2 agonist clonidine lowers blood pressure); (2) 5-hydroxytryptamine (5-HT, also called serotonin), which acts in the brain and spinal cord to inhibit preganglionic sympathetic neurons; and (3) angiotensin II, which acts in the hypothalamus to stimulate sympathetic outflow.

REFLEX BEHAVIOR OF THE CARDIOVASCULAR SYSTEM

The most important reflex behavior of the cardiovascular system originates in the stretch receptors[4] located in various blood vessels and in the atria. The receptors are positioned in the walls of these tissues in such a way that volume increases within the lumen stretch the receptors along with the rest of the wall. Because of the high compliance of the atria, large volume changes are accompanied by relatively small pressure changes, and the stretch receptors are often called *volume receptors*. Stretch receptors in the arteries, where compliance is lower, are called *pressure receptors* or *baroreceptors* because small changes in volume accompany relatively large changes in pressure.

BARORECEPTOR REFLEX
The *carotid sinus* and *aortic baroreceptors* are exceedingly important in the rapid, short-term regulation of arterial blood pressure. The carotid sinus is a slight dilation of the internal carotid artery located near its origin above the bifurcation of the common carotid artery. Baroreceptors are located in the wall of the carotid sinus. The aortic baroreceptors are located in the wall of the arch of the aorta, where they function very much like the carotid sinus baroreceptors. The carotid sinus baroreceptors have been studied in greater detail because they are more accessible experimentally, and their effects

---

[4]These receptors are not related to the neurotransmitter receptors discussed earlier. Stretch receptors are cells that respond to stretch by depolarizing, whereas the transmitter receptors are proteins that bind the neurotransmitter and initiate cellular effects.

on the medullary cardiovascular center will be emphasized here. The afferent nerve fibers from these receptors run to both the medullary cardiovascular center and to higher areas of the brain.

Increased pressure in the carotid sinus stretches the carotid sinus baroreceptors, which in turn increases their firing rate. The increased action potential traffic to the medullary cardiovascular center subsequently increases the parasympathetic neural activity to the heart and decreases the sympathetic neural activity to the heart and resistance vessels (primarily arterioles) (fig. 5-6). These changes in neural activity result in a decrease in resistance. Since $\bar{P}_a$ = $TPR \times \dot{Q}$, mean arterial pressure is returned toward the control value. This completes a negative feedback loop by which increases in the mean arterial pressure can be attenuated. Conversely, decreases in carotid sinus pressure (and decreased stretch of the baroreceptors) increase sympathetic and decrease parasympathetic neural activity, resulting in increased heart rate, stroke volume, and TPR, and a return in blood pressure toward control. With pronounced falls in mean arterial pressure, an increase in

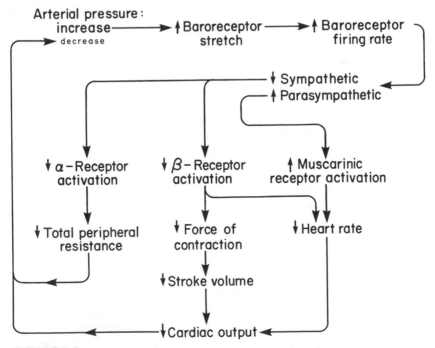

FIGURE 5-6.
Effect of the baroreceptor reflex on increased arterial pressure.

sympathetic neural activity to veins occurs. This causes contraction of the venous smooth muscle and reduces venous compliance. The decreased venous compliance shifts blood toward the central blood volume, increasing right atrial pressure and, in turn, stroke volume (chapter 3).

Not all vascular beds are equally affected by the sympathetic neural discharge initiated by the baroreceptor reflex. For example, brain and coronary arteries are less affected than skeletal muscle, splanchnic, or cutaneous arteries. Brain blood flow apparently decreases only a small amount, and coronary blood flow actually increases (despite the increased sympathetic vasoconstrictor activity) owing to the increased metabolic activity of the heart caused by the increased heart rate and stroke volume (see chapter 7). Because of this differential effect, the maintenance of blood pressure by the baroreceptor reflex does not interfere appreciably with the blood supply to the two most vital organs: the heart and the brain.

The effective range of the arterial baroreceptor mechanism (fig. 5-7) is from 40 mmHg (where the receptors stop firing) to approximately 180 mmHg (where the firing rate reaches a maximum). The firing rate of the baroreceptors increases with pulse pressure for a given mean arterial pressure.

An important property of the baroreceptor is that it adapts over a period of one or two days to the prevailing mean arterial pressure. Consequently, if the mean arterial pressure is artificially held at an elevated level, the tendency for a decrease in cardiac output and total peripheral resistance due to the baroreceptor reflex will disappear rather quickly, perhaps within 24 hours. In part, this occurs because the presence of sustained hypertension causes a reduction in the rate of baroreceptor firing for a given mean arterial pressure (fig. 5-7). This is an example of receptor adaptation. There is also a "resetting" of the reflex within the central nervous system. Consequently, the baroreceptor mechanism is the "first line of defense" in the maintenance of normal blood pressure (and makes possible the rapid control of blood pressure needed with changes in posture and exercise), but it cannot provide the long-term control of blood pressure needed from week to week and month to month.

VOLUME RECEPTOR REFLEX

The atrial stretch (volume) receptors are located at the junction of the atria and the great veins emptying into them, that is, the vena

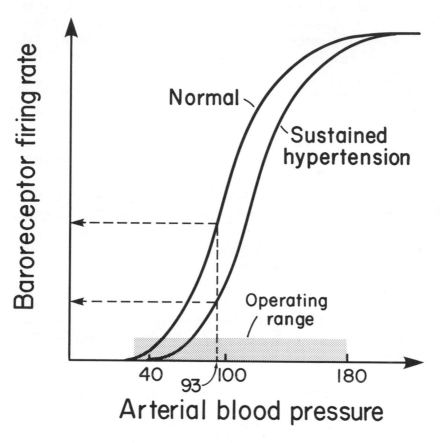

FIGURE 5-7.
Baroreceptor nerve firing rate as a function of arterial blood pressure.

cavae in the case of the right atrium and the pulmonary veins in the case of the left atrium. These receptors increase their firing rate when the volume of the atria increases and when the atria contract. The afferent fibers arising from these receptors, along with those of the aortic baroreceptors, travel in the vagus nerve to the medulla. The atrial volume receptors project to the medullary cardiovascular center, as do the arterial baroreceptors. Stretching of the atrial receptors likewise results in increased sympathetic neural activity to the SA node (increased heart rate) and decreased sympathetic activity to the kidneys (fig. 5-8). These atrial volume receptors also project to the hypothalamus, where release of vasopressin is controlled. Vasopressin causes the kidney to retain water and initiates an in-

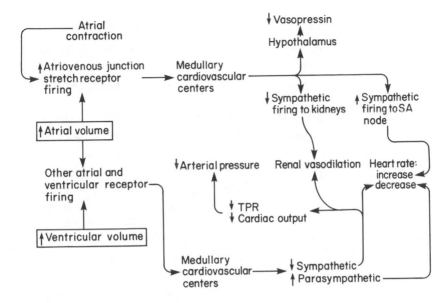

FIGURE 5-8.
Effect of increased atrial and ventricular volume on the cardiovascular system. Stretching of volume receptors causes renal vasodilation and decreased vasopressin secretion. It also causes peripheral vasodilation and decreased ventricular contractility. Effects on heart rate are variable because of conflicting effects between atriovenous junction receptors and other receptors distributed throughout the atria and ventricles.

crease in blood volume, as will be discussed later. Increased stretch of atrial receptors results in decreased vasopressin release, diuresis, and increased heart rate. The diuresis tends to decrease blood volume. Both the increased heart rate and decreased blood volume lower atrial volume and reduce stretch. This completes a negative feedback loop.

Other stretch receptors in the atria and ventricles have the same effect as arterial baroreceptors; an increase in stretch causes an increase in parasympathetic outflow and a decrease in sympathetic outflow, and a fall in blood pressure.

In summary, increased central blood volume increases the firing of stretch receptors in the heart. This input to the medullary cardiovascular neurons causes decreased sympathetic output to blood vessels, reducing total peripheral resistance. The effect on heart rate is more variable because stretch of some receptors leads to an increase and stretch of others to a decrease in heart rate. The overall effect is that stretching of volume receptors tends to reinforce the actions caused by stretching of baroreceptors.

CHEMORECEPTOR REFLEX

Another reflex pathway begins with excitation of the *chemoreceptors,* which are located peripherally in the *carotid* and *aortic bodies,* or centrally in the medulla. The carotid and aortic bodies are specialized structures located in approximately the same areas as the carotid and aortic baroreceptors. They are primarily sensitive to elevated pCO_2 and decreased pH and pO_2. The peripheral chemoreceptors exhibit increased firing rate when (1) the pO_2 of the arterial blood is low, (2) pCO_2 or H^+ concentration of arterial blood is increased, (3) the flow through the bodies is very low or stopped, or (4) a chemical is given that blocks oxidative metabolism in the chemoreceptor cells. The central medullary chemoreceptors increase their firing rate primarily in response to elevated pCO_2 and H^+ concentration. The increased firing of both peripheral and central chemoreceptors leads, via reflex pathways through the medullary cardiovascular center, to profound peripheral vasoconstriction as well as increased heart rate and cardiac output. The blood pressure is markedly elevated. If respiratory movements are voluntarily stopped the vasoconstriction is even more intense, but a striking bradycardia and decreased cardiac output occur. This is part of the *diving response* and is discussed later. As is the case of the baroreceptor reflex, the coronary and cerebral circulation are not subjected to the same degree of vasoconstrictor effects and exhibit vasodilation due to local metabolic effects.

Chemoreceptor drive is probably quite important in the cardiovascular response to hemorrhagic hypotension. As blood pressure falls, blood flow through the carotid and aortic bodies decreases and chemoreceptor neural firing increases. This occurs because the decrease in blood flow lowers the pO_2 of these chemoreceptors.

OTHER REFLEXES

Reflex cardiovascular responses to pain also occur. Two different responses to pain may be seen. In the first and most common reaction, pain causes an increased sympathetic activity to the heart and blood vessels coupled with a decreased parasympathetic activity to the heart. These events lead to increases in cardiac output, total peripheral resistance, and mean arterial pressure. An example of this reaction is the elevated blood pressure that normally occurs when an extremity is placed in ice water. This is called the *cold pressor response,* and the increase in blood pressure produced by this challenge is exaggerated in some forms of hypertension. A second type of response is produced by deep pain. Here, the stimulation of deep pain fibers associated with crushing injuries, disruption of joints, testicular trauma, or distention of the abdominal organs results in diminished sympathetic neural activity and enhanced parasympathetic activity, with decreased cardiac output and TPR and a drop in blood pressure. This hypotensive response contributes to certain forms of shock. Injection of 5-hydroxytryptamine or certain alkaloids into the coronary arteries supplying posterior regions of the ventricles causes reflex bradycardia and hypotension. This reflex could play a role in the cardiovascular response to myocardial infarction.

CORTICOHYPOTHALAMIC CARDIOVASCULAR PATTERNS

Corticohypothalamic response patterns are integrated in the hypothalamus, and the stimulation of certain areas of the hypothalamus leads to distinct behavioral, and cardiovascular, response patterns. An example of this is the *defense reaction.* The rage response of cats described earlier in this chapter is an exaggerated defense reaction. In general, the behavioral pattern exhibited in the defense reaction includes increased skeletal muscle tone and general alertness. This is accomplished by increased sympathetic neural activity to blood vessels. The sympathetic cholinergic fibers innervating skeletal muscle arterioles are activated, and acetylcholine is released rather than norepinephrine; this causes vasodilation in skeletal muscle. The result of this cardiovascular response is to increase (1) cardiac output (increased heart rate and stroke volume), (2) blood pressure, and (3) skeletal muscle blood flow, and to reduce flow to the splanchnic and renal vascular beds. This anticipatory redistribution of blood flow to muscle in a behavioral pattern, which involves either *"fight or flight,"* may provide an all-important competitive edge in lower animals where split seconds separate the survivors from those less fortunate. Emotional situations often bring on the defense reaction in civilized people, but it is usually not accompanied by the muscle exercise that would follow in the more primitive situations. Much current speculation centers on the question whether the dissociation of the cardiovascular component of the defense reaction from the behavioral component ("fight or flight") is deleterious.

Vasovagal syncope ("fainting") is the somatic and cardiovascular response to certain emotional experiences. Stimulation of specific areas of the cerebral cortex can lead to the sudden relaxation of skeletal muscles, depression of respiration, and loss of consciousness. The cardiovascular events accompanying these somatic changes include profound parasympathetic bradycardia and removal of sympathetic vasoconstrictor tone (with a dramatic drop in heart rate, cardiac output, and total peripheral resistance). The resultant decrease in mean arterial pressure results in unconsciousness because of lowered cerebral blood flow. Vasovagal syncope appears in lower animals as the "playing dead" response so typical of the opossum.

The cardiovascular response associated with embarrassment *(blushing)* is an increase in skin blood flow, which follows the sudden removal of the normal level of sympathetic vasoconstrictor activity.

The cardiovascular response to *diving* is observed best in seals and ducks, but is also present in humans. An experienced diver exhibits intense slowing of the heart (parasympathetic) and peripheral vasoconstriction (sympathetic) when his or her face is submerged. During the dive this is reinforced by the chemoreceptor reflex which, in the absence of respiratory movements, causes the same cardiovascular response. The arterioles of the brain and the heart are not constricted; therefore the (minimal) cardiac output is distributed to those organs. This heart-brain circuit makes use of the oxygen stored in the blood that would normally be used by the other tissues, especially skeletal muscle. Once the diver surfaces, the heart rate and cardiac output increase dramatically and the peripheral vasoconstriction is replaced by vasodilation, restoring nutrient flow to wash out accumulated waste products.

A change in the *temperature* of the thermoregulatory hypothalamic neurons induces dramatic changes in skin blood flow. This is accomplished by selective adjustment of the sympathetic activity to the skin. Sympathetic activity to other organs does not necessarily change. There is no clearly demonstrated cutaneous neural vasodilator system. As the hypothalamus is heated, sympathetic vasoconstrictor activity decreases, allowing increased blood flow through skin and increased heat dissipation. Further increases in hypothalamic temperature result in increased sweat gland activity, which causes increased skin blood flow (as is discussed in chapter 7). The vasodilation in response to increased sweat gland activity can raise blood flow above the level produced by total withdrawal of sympathetic neural activity alone.

Stimulation of certain parts of the hypothalamus, as well as other parts of the brain, initiates the complete behavioral pattern associated with *copulation,* including vasodilation and erection of the genital organs. Males who have disruption or transection of the spinal cord can still achieve erection by tactile stimulation of the genital organs; thus it is likely that vasodilation of the genitalia results from a spinal reflex that is normally influenced by neural input from the cortical and hypothalamic areas. Sacral parasympathetic fibers are responsible for the vasodilation that initiates erection.

Several of the corticohypothalamic responses, including the defense reaction, cause mean arterial pressure to rise above normal despite the fact that heart rate and cardiac output are also increased. How can this happen if the baroreceptor reflex is working? In these circumstances the interconnections between the hypothalamus and medullary areas inhibit the baroreceptor reflex and allow the corticohypothalamic response to predominate. The various cardiovascular response patterns do not necessarily occur in isolation as we have described them. Many of them interact, reflecting the extensive neural interconnections at all levels of the central nervous system. For example, the defense reaction plays a role in the cardiovascular events associated with diving.

Cardiovascular responses can be conditioned (as can other autonomic responses, e.g., those observed in Pavlov's famous experiments). Both classical and operant conditioning techniques have been used to raise and lower the blood pressure and heart rate of animals. Humans can also be taught to alter their heart rate and blood pressure by using a variety of behavioral techniques (e.g., biofeedback). Therapeutic implications of the behavioral control of various cardiovascular events are enormous.

HORMONAL CONTROL SYSTEM

ADRENAL MEDULLA

When the sympathetic nervous system is activated, the adrenal medulla releases epinephrine and norepinephrine into the blood. Changes in the circulating levels of epinephrine and norepinephrine have relatively little effect when compared with the direct release of norepinephrine from nerve endings nestled close to the target cells. Increased circulating epinephrine causes skeletal muscle vasodilation during the defense reaction. In this situation epinephrine binds to β_2-receptors of skeletal muscle arterioles and causes vasodilation. Denervated organs, such as transplanted hearts, are dramatically influenced by circulating levels of epinephrine and norepinephrine. The increased sensitivity to neurotransmitters occurring in denervated organs is referred to as *denervation hypersensitivity.* Sympathetic nerves actively take up norepinephrine and epinephrine. When they are absent, more transmitter is available for binding to receptors. (This, however, is not the only mechanism responsible for denervation hypersensitivity; other factors, such as an increase in the number of adrenergic receptors in the target tissue, may be involved.) Circulating levels of norepinephrine and epinephrine increase with exercise, and because of denervation hypersensitivity, transplanted hearts are able to perform almost as well as normal hearts.

VASOPRESSIN

Vasopressin[5] is released by the posterior pituitary gland under the control of the hypothalamus. The three important classes of stimuli leading to vasopressin release are (1) increased plasma osmolarity; (2) decreased atrial stretch receptor firing; and (3) various sorts of stress, such as physical injury or surgery. Vasopressin is a vasoconstrictor, but it is not ordinarily present in the plasma in high enough concentration to exert much direct effect on blood vessels. It exerts its major effect on the cardiovascular system by causing the retention of water by the kidneys. This is an important part of the neurohumoral mechanisms that regulate blood volume. Vasopressin is also a potent vasoconstrictor, and it probably contributes to increased total peripheral resistance when it is elevated in response to a diminished blood volume.

RENIN-ANGIOTENSIN-ALDOSTERONE SYSTEM

A variety of stimuli cause release of *renin* from the kidney. This hormone is an enzyme that catalyzes the conversion of angiotensinogen, a plasma protein, to angiotensin I. Angiotensin I is then

---

[5]Vasopressin (and the hormone systems that remain to be discussed) are usually considered to be in the province of the renal physiologist. Modern concepts regarding the control of the cardiovascular system are so dependent upon a knowledge of the regulation of salt and water balance that a discussion of these hormone systems has been included in this text. Only those points essential for an understanding of cardiovascular function have been mentioned. You should consult a text on renal physiology for more information on these hormonal systems and their effects on the kidney.

converted to angiotensin II by *converting enzyme.* Angiotensin II is a powerful arterial constrictor. In some circumstances it is present in plasma in concentrations high enough to cause vasoconstriction and influence peripheral resistance. Angiotensin also causes the release of aldosterone from the adrenal cortex. One of the effects of aldosterone is to reduce renal excretion of Na^+, the major cation of the extracellular fluid. Retention of Na^+ paves the way for increasing blood volume. Factors that control renin release, and therefore angiotensin and aldosterone levels, are (1) the amount of Na^+ presented to the distal tubules of the kidney; (2) stretch of small arterioles of the kidney; and (3) activation of β-receptors of the cells that store renin in the kidney, the *juxtaglomerular* cells. These controls usually operate synergistically in their effect on renin release (fig. 5-9). For example, a decrease in mean arterial pressure results in an increase in sympathetic α-adrenergic constriction of renal arteries.

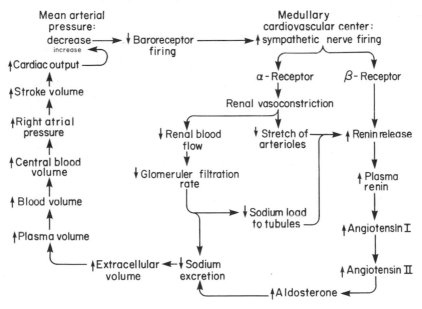

FIGURE 5-9.
Effect of decrease in mean arterial pressure on sodium excretion.

This vasoconstriction decreases the stretch of the small arterioles, which results in the release of renin. The decreased renal blood flow is accompanied by a fall in the glomerular filtration rate and a decrease in the mass of Na^+ presented to the distal tubule, which also stimulates renin release. The sympathetic neural activity not only causes vasoconstriction, but also initiates the release of renin by directly stimulating the juxtaglomerular cells. Thus increased renal sympathetic neural activity stimulates renin release, and decreased sympathetic neural activity to the kidney usually results in reduced renin release.

ERYTHROPOIETIN

Erythropoietin is another hormone produced by the kidney; it causes the bone marrow to increase production of red blood cells, thus increasing the total mass of red cells. The stimuli for increased erythropoietin release include hypoxia and anemia. If vasopressin and aldosterone secretion are increased, salt and water retention is enhanced, which results in an increase in plasma volume. The increased plasma volume in the face of a constant red blood cell volume results in a lower hematocrit. The decrease in hematocrit stimulates erythropoietin release; this increases red blood cell synthesis and red cell mass, and therefore balances the increase in plasma volume caused by aldosterone and vasopressin. Thus aldosterone, vasopressin, and erythropoietin are the hormonal basis for the control of blood volume. Changing the total blood volume leads to changes in the central blood volume (assuming that distribution of blood volume remains constant). Control of total blood volume, central venous volume, and cardiac output are extremely important in the long-term regulation of blood pressure.

ATRIAL NATRIURETIC PEPTIDE (ANP)

This polypeptide is synthesized and stored in the atrial muscle cells and is released into the bloodstream when the atria are stretched. It increases the glomerular filtration rate and promotes Na^+ excretion. ANP may be partially responsible for the reduction in blood flow that occurs in weightlessness or bed rest (see chapter 8).

Suggested Readings

Berne RM, Levy MN (eds.): *Cardiovascular Physiology.* 4th ed. St. Louis, The C. V. Mosby Company, 1981, pp 123-181
Guyton AC: *Textbook of Medical Physiology.* 6th ed. Philadelphia, W.B. Saunders Co., 1981, pp 246-272
Heymans CJF, Folkow B: Vasomotor control and the regulation of blood pressure. In *Circulation of the Blood: Men and Ideas.* Edited by AP Fishman and DW Richards. Bethesda, American Physiological Society, 1982, 407-486

Korner PI: Central nervous control of autonomic cardiovascular function. In *Handbook of Physiology. Section 2. The Cardiovascular System.* Edited by RM Berne, N Sperelakis, SR Geiger. Bethesda, American Physiological Society, 1979, vol. 1, pp 641-740

Shepherd JT, Vanhoutte PM (eds.): *The Human Cardiovascular System.* New York, Raven Press, 1979, pp 107-144, 180-207

Valtin H: *Renal Function: Mechanisms Preserving Fluid and Solute Balance in Health.* Boston, Little Brown and Co., 1973

Vander AT: *Renal Physiology.* 2d ed. New York, McGraw-Hill, 1980

Chapter 6

Regulation of Flow and Exchange

Chapters 6 and 7 describe the regulation of blood flow and microvascular exchange in the various tissues of the body. This chapter deals with the components of the blood vessel wall, with special emphasis on the two functionally unique cells of the vascular wall, endothelial cells and vascular myocytes. It also deals with the principles of microvascular exchange.

FUNCTIONAL ANATOMY

As the vascular tree branches, the anatomy and function of successive segments change. Figure 6-1 shows the basic structural features of each of the successive segments of the systemic circulation. Large arteries, like the aorta, have a thick wall that contains concentric elastic laminae in the media. These vessels dampen pulsations in pressure and flow arising from the cyclical pumping of the heart. They do this by expanding during systole and recoiling during diastole. The medium-sized muscular arteries have a higher proportion of muscle as compared with elastic tissue in their media. These vessels can offer a variable resistance to flow by contraction or relaxation of the muscle. Arterioles (20-200 μm in diameter) contain from one to several layers of smooth muscle and little else in their media. They are capable of dramatic changes in diameter and are the main site for regulation of vascular resistance. Smaller branches, *metarterioles*, have an interrupted layer of smooth muscle. *Capillaries* may arise from either metarterioles or small arterioles. The walls of capillaries are composed of flat endothelial cells with virtually no connective tissue and no smooth muscle. They are typically 0.5 to 1 mm in length and 5 μm in diameter. In most tissues, capillaries form a network through which red blood cells must squeeze in order to reach the small venules distal to the capillaries. The walls

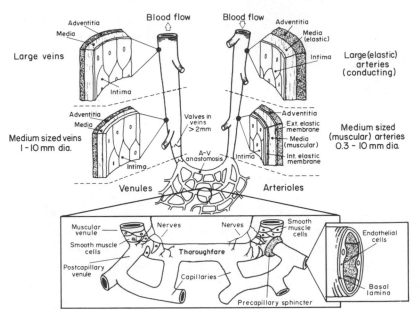

FIGURE 6-1.
Structural features of various segments of the vascular tree.

of the venules are likewise nothing more than endothelium surrounded by a basement membrane and a scant amount of connective tissue. Because the walls of capillaries and venules are so thin, an
exchange of substances between interstitial fluid and blood occurs
across them.

In some tissues, a precapillary sphincter encircles the entrance
to each capillary. This ring of smooth muscle can open or close, thus
determining whether or not the capillary is perfused by blood. In
other tissues, such as skeletal muscle, precapillary sphincters do not
exist as specific entities; it is thought that the final portions of metar-
teriolar smooth muscle may play the same role in opening and closing capillaries. In many tissues (including gut, muscle, and
myocardium), not all capillaries are open at the same time. Instead,
capillaries open and close in what appears to be a random fashion,
and only a fraction of the total number of capillaries is available for
exchange of nutrients and waste products with flowing blood at any
given moment. For example, in resting skeletal muscle only one-
fourth to one-third of all capillaries are open at any given time. During vigorous exercise all of the capillaries may be open
concurrently, thereby increasing the total capillary surface area for
exchange by several-fold.

When observed under the microscope, red blood cells in most capillaries stop and start intermittently. A few capillaries appear to be preferential routes, and there is usually a steady stream of red cells through these *thoroughfare channels*. Red blood cells must squeeze through capillaries one at a time, because capillaries are only 4-5 μm in diameter whereas human red cells have a diameter of roughly 7 μm. As red cells enter the capillaries, they must change from their normal discoid shape to the shape of a parachute (with the middle of the cell leading and the edges trailing behind). This requires tremendous resiliency on the part of each red cell. Diseases that increase the fragility of the red cell membrane (e.g., sickle-cell anemia) greatly enhance the chance that cells will be damaged as they cross the capillary bed. It appears that certain pharmacologic agents (e.g., pentoxifylline) exert their viscosity-reducing effects by enhancing the flexibility of the red blood cell membrane.

The vascular beds of some tissues, for example, skin, have *arteriovenous anastomoses* (AV shunts). These blood vessels have larger lumens than capillaries and contain smooth muscle. They may be open or closed depending upon the tone of the smooth muscle. If the arteriovenous anastomoses are open, they form low-resistance preferential channels that divert flow from the capillary bed (see fig. 6-1). Thus not all blood flow through the microcirculation of a tissue need be *nutrient* blood flow.

Medium-sized veins have a continuous layer of smooth muscle and well-defined connective tissue support in the adventitia. As discussed in Chapter 4, these veins are very compliant and can change capacity by contraction and relaxation of their smooth muscle. Large veins have a thick wall made up primarily of connective tissue, with some smooth muscle.

ENDOTHELIAL CELLS
Endothelial cells line the entire vascular tree. These are flat cells approximately 0.2-0.5 μm thick. Substances must pass through or between endothelial cells to gain access to the subendothelial region of the blood vessel wall, or interstitial space in the case of capillaries and venules. There are a number of pathways for transport between and through endothelial cells. These pathways include tight junctions, intercellular clefts, and pinocytotic vesicles (fig. 6-2). Most connections between endothelial cells on the arterial side of the circulation are tight junctions, with occasional intercellular clefts.

A.

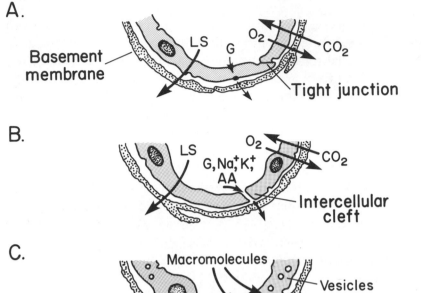

B.

C.

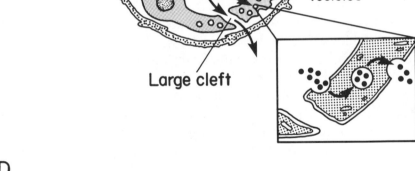

D.

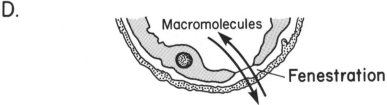

FIGURE 6-2.
Pathways for microvascular transport. (A) Brain capillary, in which tight junctions join endothelial cells. Lipid soluble substances (LS) including gases diffuse through plasma membranes. Hydrophilic substances depend upon carrier proteins in plasma membranes, as does glucose (G). (B) Muscle capillary, in which hydrophilic substances (AA = amino acids) can diffuse through clefts between endothelial cells. (C) Small venule from muscle, in which there are large clefts and pinocytotic vesicles, both of which transport macromolecules, for example, plasma proteins. (D) Fenestrated capillary (as occurs in glands), in which there are large gaps containing a thin membrane. Macromolecules, for example, protein hormones, can diffuse through the fenestrations.

There are also numerous pinocytotic vesicles. The venous side of the circulation contains large intercellular clefts.

Endothelial cells subserve many important functions aside from being a physical lining for the blood vessel wall. They are the elements of the vascular wall that prevent intravascular clotting (the clotting phenomenon has already been discussed in Chapter 1). Endothelial cells prevent the initiation of platelet aggregation by releasing *prostacyclin*, a metabolite of arachidonic acid. Endothelial cells are also involved in the metabolism of a large number of substances found in plasma. This has been well studied in the lung and will be described in Chapter 7. Finally, endothelial cells influence the contraction of vascular smooth muscle. A number of substances found in plasma are capable of indirectly influencing smooth muscle contraction by an effect on endothelial cells.

VASCULAR SMOOTH MUSCLE

The other major cellular component of the vessel wall is *vascular smooth muscle*. These cells are long (50-100 μm) and thin (5 μm), and they encircle the lumen. The regulation of their contractile activity bears many similarities to cardiac muscle, but is different enough to warrant some description:

Excitation

Unlike cardiac muscle, vascular smooth muscle has resting tone. That is, it exerts a certain level of contractile force under basal conditions. Sometimes this tone is *myogenic* (originating in the muscle itself), and in other cases it results from the influence of nerves or circulating vasoactive agents. A wide variety of stimuli influence resting tone, some causing relaxation and others contraction. Most of these agents bind to a membrane receptor and exert an effect on contractile proteins by means of a second messenger.

The *membrane potential* of vascular myocytes is determined by the relative permeabilities of the plasma membrane to K^+, Na^+, and Ca^{2+} and by the *electrogenic* activity of the Na^+, K^+ pump (Na^+, K^+-ATPase). The resting membrane potential of a typical vascular myocyte is -50 to -60 mV. This potential is primarily the result of the high permeability of the plasma membrane to K^+ relative to Na^+ and Ca^{2+}. However, in vascular myocytes there is a much greater leak of K^+ and Na^+ across the membrane at rest than in cardiac muscle. Therefore the Na^+, K^+ pump must have a much higher activity to maintain concentration differences of the two cations across the plasma membrane. Because three Na^+ are exchanged for every two K^+, the pump causes a net flux of positive charge out of the cell and makes the membrane potential more negative by approximately 10 mV. That is, of a resting membrane potential of -60 mV, -50 mV is contributed by K^+ leak channels and -10 mV by the Na^+,K^+ pump.

When the membrane is depolarized, more Ca^{2+} enters the vascular myocyte and contraction results. When the cell is hyperpolarized, less Ca^{2+} enters and the cell relaxes. Vasoactive agents can cause changes in membrane potential by (1) opening or closing cation channels or (2) stimulating or inhibiting the Na^+,K^+ pump. As in cardiac muscle, cytosolic Ca^{2+} concentration is a key factor in regulating contraction of the vascular myocyte. However, vascular myocytes are more dependent upon extracellular Ca^{2+} to raise cytosolic Ca^{2+} concentration than is cardiac muscle.

Contraction

Regulation of the contractile proteins, actin and myosin, is very different in vascular and cardiac myocytes. In vascular myocytes increased cytosolic Ca^{2+} binds to the intracellular protein *calmodulin*. The Ca^{2+}-calmodulin complex then binds to and activates the enzyme myosin light chain kinase. This enzyme catalyzes phosphorylation of myosin light chains and thereby initiates actin-myosin interaction and vascular myocyte contraction. The activity of myosin light chain kinase is also regulated by a cAMP-dependent kinase. This kinase phosphorylates myosin light chain kinase and reduces its activation by the Ca^{2+}-calmodulin complex (fig. 6-3).

EXCHANGE ACROSS THE CAPILLARY WALL

The capillary wall is a sheet of endothelial cells one cell layer thick, supported by a basement membrane. In most tissues, fluid-filled clefts between endothelial cells are important in determining the transport characteristics of the capillary wall because water-soluble substances pass through them. Lipid-soluble substances pass readily through the plasma membrane of the endothelial cells and are not dependent upon the clefts between cells. The water-filled clefts constitute only a small percentage ($<1\%$) of the total area of the capillary endothelium. Thus more than 100 times more area is available for diffusion of lipid-soluble substances than for water-soluble substances.

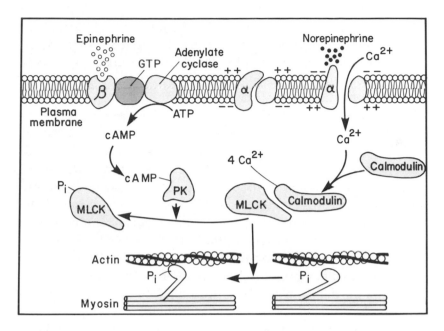

FIGURE 6-3.

Contraction of vascular smooth muscle. Contractile tone of vascular myocytes depends upon the degree of activation of myosin light chain kinase (MLCK), which catalyzes phosphorylation of myosin and promotes actin-myosin crossbridge cycling. Ca^{2+}-calmodulin complex combines with and activates myosin light chain kinase. Phosphorylation of myosin light chain kinase by a cAMP-dependent protein kinase (PK) inhibits its combination with Ca^{2+}-calmodulin complex. Norepinephrine binds to α-adrenergic receptors and opens Ca^{2+} channels, which causes Ca^{2+} entry and membrane depolarization. Epinephrine binds to β-adrenergic receptors and, via the guanine nucleotide subunit (GTP), causes activation of adenylate cyclase. This raises cAMP, activates a protein kinase, and phosphorylates myosin light chain kinase. (P_i = phosphate)

The capillary clefts, or pores,[1] vary in size from tissue to tissue. At one extreme there are no clefts between endothelial cells of brain capillaries (only tight junctions). Very small molecules such as water and urea diffuse between the plasma and the brain interstitium directly through plasma membranes (fig. 6-2A). Glucose, the primary energy substrate of brain cells, must cross the capillary endothelial plasma membranes by carrier-mediated facilitated

---

[1]The clefts between cells were called *pores* by J. R. Pappenheimer. On the basis of data on the diffusion of water-soluble molecules, he calculated an equivalent pore radius for the fluid-filled channels of skeletal muscle capillaries. He recognized that the channels might have the shape of slits or clefts, and he also calculated their size. Electron microscopists were subsequently able to verify the existence of the channels that Pappenheimer predicted. Because the prediction of the cylindrical pore radius has become a classic work in physiology, the fluid-filled channels are often referred to as pores rather than a name more suited to their anatomy.

diffusion. The selective impermeability of brain capillaries is referred to as the *blood-brain barrier.* Lipid-soluble substances have no trouble crossing the blood-brain barrier because they readily pass through the plasma membranes of endothelial cells.

An intermediate type of capillary endothelium is found in skeletal and cardiac muscle. In these tissues, the clefts between endothelial cells have a width of approximately 30-40 Å (fig. 6-2B). Channels of this size allow the passage of electrolytes, glucose, amino acids, small polypeptides, and other water-soluble substances in this size range. Plasma proteins cannot pass through these pores. Lipid-soluble substances can, of course, cross the entire capillary endothelial surface as in brain capillaries. Larger molecules, for example, plasma proteins, move from plasma to the interstitial space by a second transport system located in small venules (fig. 6-2C). This transport system has two components: first, there are a few large clefts that permit simple diffusion of plasma proteins between the two spaces; second, there are pinocytotic vesicles that engulf plasma and transport it across the cell. Protein is subsequently removed from the interstitial space by lymphatic flow.

At the other end of the spectrum are the *fenestrations* of capillary endothelium in endocrine glands, kidney, and intestine. These fenestrations are large openings (60-120 nm in diameter) through the cells that allow the passage of water-soluble molecules as large as plasma proteins (fig. 6-2D).

The extent to which the capillary wall allows certain substances to pass is referred to as the *permeability* to that substance. In general, capillary walls are much more permeable to lipid-soluble substances than to water-soluble substances, and to low-molecular weight substances than to high-molecular weight substances.

DIFFUSIONAL EXCHANGE

The quantitatively important exchange of substances involved in cell nutrition and waste removal occurs by diffusion. Diffusion to and from tissues is under physiological control because the blood flow and the number of open capillaries can be regulated by vascular smooth muscle tone. The factors affecting diffusional exchange can best be considered by using Fick's law for diffusion:

$$ds/dt = PA\,(C_p - C_t)/\Delta X.$$

The rate of solute movement in moles per second (ds/dt) is related to the permeability of the capillary to a particular solute (P), the area available for diffusion (A), the concentration difference between the plasma and tissue ($C_p - C_t$) and the path distance between the plasma and the site in tissue to or from which the solute is diffusing (ΔX). Permeability depends upon the temperature and the molecular weight of the substance (increasing with increases in temperature and decreasing with the square root of the molecular weight). Permeability also depends upon the lipid solubility of the solute, and, if the solute is hydrophilic, the size of the molecule relative to the size of pores through which it must pass. If the solute is lipid-soluble or very small relative to pore size, P is high. If the solute is hydrophilic and large, P is small.

Several of the factors in Fick's law are under physiologic control. First, the area available for diffusion can be regulated by increasing or decreasing the number of open capillaries. This is accomplished by regulating the activity of the precapillary sphincters (or their equivalents). The precapillary smooth muscle is probably not innervated and is predominantly affected by local factors such as vasodilator metabolites released from parenchymal cells (see chapter 7). Additional open capillaries give more surface area for diffusion, and this enhances the transport of O_2, CO_2 and substrates.

Second, the distance across which diffusion must occur is controlled by the number of open capillaries. As vasodilator metabolites accumulate, precapillary sphincters open and the average distance from capillaries to various tissue sites decreases (fig. 6-4).

Concentration difference is the other physiologic determinant of diffusion rates. For example, the increase in tissue production of CO_2 that accompanies increased metabolism elevates tissue CO_2 concentration and pCO_2, and increases its diffusion rate into capillaries. Flow changes are also important in determining the concentration difference. If the flow increases in the above example, the CO_2 concentration of the capillary blood will remain lower throughout the capillary and therefore enhance the concentration difference, which raises the diffusion rate. Conversely, if oxygen consumption increases, the tissue pO_2 falls and a more rapid diffusion of oxygen from the capillary into the tissue occurs. If flow subsequently increases, the oxygen concentration of the blood is held at a higher level along the length of the capillary; this increases the concentration difference and raises the diffusion rate of oxygen into the tissue (fig. 6-5).

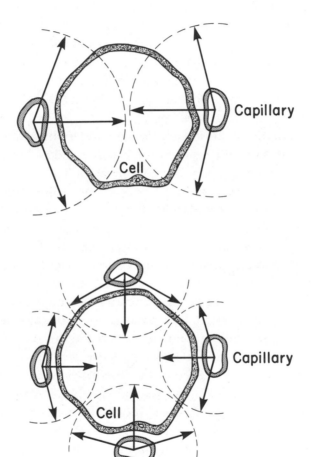

FIGURE 6-4.
Capillary diffusion distances. The effect of opening more capillaries on diffusion distance is indicated by the length of the arrows.

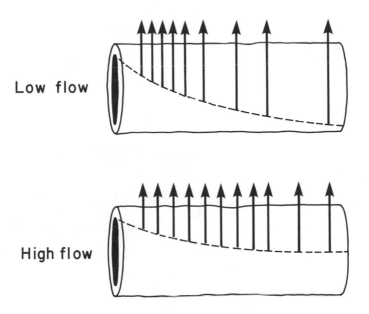

FIGURE 6-5.
Effect of flow on capillary pO_2 and diffusion of O_2 into tissue. The dashed line inside the capillary represents the pO_2 along the capillary, and the density of the arrows the diffusion of O_2.

In summary, the physiologically controlled elements of Fick's law are (1) the surface area for diffusion (by number of open capillaries), (2) diffusion distance (also by number of open capillaries), and (3) concentration differences (by alteration in tissue or blood concentration and blood flow). Increased metabolic needs of tissues are met by changing all three of these factors. Figure 6-6 shows how relaxation of vascular smooth muscle by local vasodilator factors can result in changes that influence capillary diffusion.

CAPILLARY FILTRATION AND REABSORPTION

Water and water-soluble solutes move readily between the plasma and the interstitial space through pores in capillary membranes (except brain capillaries). The forces that govern the movement of flu-

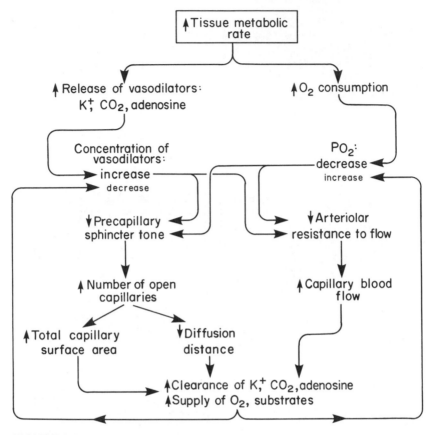

FIGURE 6-6.
Relationship between tissue metabolic rate and factors affecting capillary transport.

ids and solutes across capillary walls are of tremendous importance because their balance determines the volume of the plasma relative to the interstitial fluid. If a large fraction of plasma were to enter the interstitial fluid space (as occurs in some injuries, e.g., burns), blood volume would decrease and this could cause a fall in arterial pressure. The factors that determine the movement of fluid across the capillary walls are summarized in the following equation:

$$F = K_F(P_c - P_i + \pi_i - \pi_c)^*$$

This equation states that the hydrostatic pressure (P_c) inside the

*This equation expresses the Starling-Landis equilibrium. Starling measured the colloid osmotic pressure of plasma and predicted that capillary pressure must balance against it. His hypothesis was tested and found to be valid 30 years later by a medical student at the University of Pennsylvania, Eugene Landis.

capillary and the colloid osmotic pressure of the interstitial space (π_i) tend to force fluid from the capillary, whereas the colloid osmotic pressure inside the capillary (π_c) and the hydrostatic pressure in the interstitial space (P_i) tend to force fluid into the capillary. The movement of fluid out of the capillary is called *filtration (F)* and movement into the capillary is called *reabsorption (−F)*. The rate of filtration that occurs in response to the differences between these pressures is determined by the capillary *filtration coefficient, K_F*. This coefficient expresses the ease with which an ultrafiltrate of plasma (primarily water and electrolytes) can pass back and forth through the capillary membrane given a certain pressure difference. K_F is a function of capillary permeability and surface area. Thus in conditions (such as exercise) when a larger number of capillaries are open, there is a greater tendency for filtration to occur given a particular pressure difference.

Mean capillary hydrostatic pressure *(P_c)* is between 8 and 25 mmHg, depending upon the particular vascular bed and the estimate used (see below). P_c is determined by (1) mean arterial pressure, (2) venous pressure, and (3) resistance to blood flow on each side of the capillary. Figure 6-7 shows how each of these variables affects capillary hydrostatic pressure. The figure demonstrates the effects of mean arterial pressure, venous pressure, and resistance on capillary hydrostatic pressure in a hypothetical skeletal muscle bed with a flow of 1 L/min. Arterial (precapillary) resistance is 0.074 PRU, and therefore the capillary pressure at the arterial end of the capillary is 26 mmHg (panel A). Capillary resistance to flow causes a pressure drop of 16 mmHg along the capillary, so mean capillary hydrostatic pressure halfway down the capillary is 18 mmHg. The venous resistance causes a pressure drop of 10 mmHg. If mean arterial pressure is raised by 50 mmHg (panel B), flow increases proportionately and the capillary hydrostatic pressure increases 9 mmHg, or approximately 20% of the increase in mean arterial pressure. Raising venous pressure 50 mmHg (panel C) decreases flow and causes a 41 mmHg rise in capillary hydrostatic pressure, which is approximately 80% of the increase in venous pressure. Thus changes in hydrostatic pressure from the venous end influence capillary hydrostatic pressure much more than do changes from the arterial end. Arteriolar vasodilation that lowers arterial resistance to one-half (panel D) increases flow 60%, and capillary hydrostatic pressure rises by 11 mmHg. Arteriolar constriction lowers flow

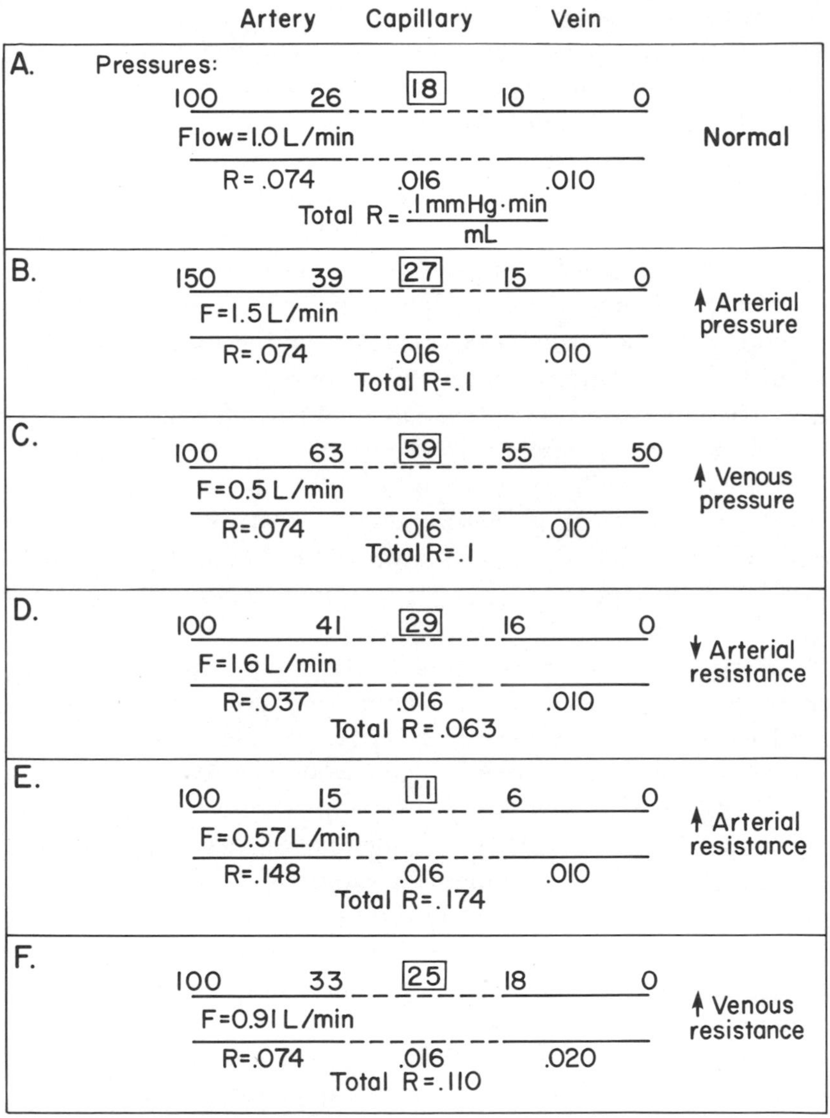

FIGURE 6-7.
Pressure differences, flow, and hydrostatic pressure in the capillaries. Note the effect of increased arterial (B) and venous (C) pressure, decreased (D) and increased (E) arterial resistance, and increased venous resistance (F) on mean capillary hydrostatic pressure. All the numbers needed to verify the calculations are provided. Going through the calculations will help clarify the role of pressure and resistance in determining capillary hydrostatic pressure.

(panel E) and lowers capillary hydrostatic pressure. Elevating venous resistance, as might happen with partial occlusion of venous drainage, elevates capillary hydrostatic pressure (panel F).

The following points should be noted from this example. (1) Increasing either arterial or venous pressure alone increases capillary hydrostatic pressure, but increasing venous pressure has a greater effect on capillary hydrostatic pressure than does increasing arterial pressure. This happens because less vascular resistance is interposed between the veins and capillaries than between the arteries and capillaries. (2) Decreasing arteriolar resistance raises capillary hydrostatic pressure by permitting a greater fraction of the arterial pressure to reach the capillaries. Increasing arteriolar resistance has the opposite effect. (3) Decreasing venous resistance lowers capillary hydrostatic pressure because less pressure drop is needed to move the blood from the capillaries to the right atrium. Increasing venous resistance likewise raises capillary hydrostatic pressure.

The hydrostatic pressure in the interstitial space (P_i) opposes the hydrostatic pressure of the plasma. This pressure is determined by the volume of fluid in the interstitial space and the compliance of the structures surrounding this space. Figure 6-8 shows the relationship between the interstitial fluid pressure and volume. The absolute value of the interstitial hydrostatic pressure is difficult to determine, and estimates range from 0 mmHg with respect to average atmospheric pressure (i.e., equal to atmospheric pressure) to − 7 mmHg (i.e., 7 mmHg less than atmospheric pressure). Most investigators agree that the hydrostatic pressure difference between capillary and interstitial space is approximately 25 mmHg. Capillary and interstitial fluid hydrostatic pressure can be estimated by a variety of techniques, and the numbers obtained by different techniques vary enough so that individual researchers can always find a set of numbers to match their prejudices. We will assume that interstitial hydrostatic pressure is subatmospheric, and will therefore use a capillary hydrostatic pressure of 18 mmHg and an interstitial hydrostatic pressure of − 7 mmHg as representative values.

As fluid filters from capillaries into the interstitial space, interstitial volume and pressure increase (fig. 6-8). The increase in interstitial pressure opposes further filtration by reducing the hydrostatic pressure gradient from capillary to interstitial fluid. As fluid is reabsorbed from the interstitial space, interstitial pressure decreases and filtration resumes.

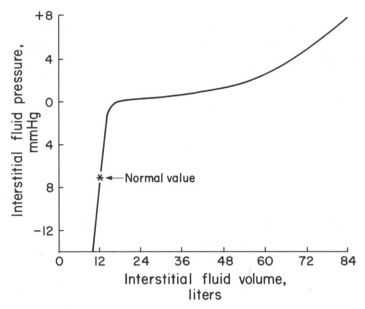

FIGURE 6-8.
Pressure-volume curve for the interstitial space. Note that the normal value for interstitial pressure is negative with respect to atmospheric pressure, and that small changes in interstitial volume cause relatively large changes in pressure in the normal range.

Colloid osmotic pressure is the other determinant of fluid balance across the capillary wall. Because the membrane is permeable to electrolytes, the greater than 5000 mmHg of osmotic pressure offered by electrolytes does not contribute to the osmotic pressure difference across the capillary membrane.[2] Only plasma proteins, which cannot pass easily across the capillary membrane, can generate an osmotic pressure gradient. The osmotic pressure developed by the protein is called the *colloid osmotic pressure.* Plasma colloid osmotic pressure is approximately 25 mmHg. The colloid pressure is caused by albumin (approximately 15 mmHg), and globulins plus other proteins (approximately 10 mmHg). The relationship between protein concentration and colloid osmotic pressure is shown in fig. 6-9. The plasma protein concentration is determined by the amount of protein present in the plasma and the volume of the plasma. The loss of large amounts of water and electrolytes (such as those produced by diarrhea, excessive sweating, or renal loss) increases the concentration of plasma proteins and therefore

[2]This point cannot be emphasized too much. Or can it? My professor of physiology fired a cannon in the lecture hall to emphasize the point. All that most of us could remember was the smell of gunpowder and, of course, that professor—for life! H. V. S.

increases the plasma colloid osmotic pressure. The increase in plasma colloid osmotic pressure subsequently draws water and electrolytes from the interstitial space into the plasma.

The colloid osmotic pressure in the interstitial space is determined by the protein concentration in this fluid (approximately 1 g/100 mL). Figure 6-9 shows that this concentration of protein will

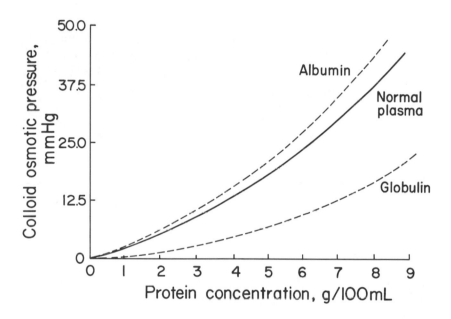

FIGURE 6-9.
Relationship between protein concentration and colloid osmotic pressure. Because the molecular weight of albumin is less than that of globulin, a given weight of albumin exerts a greater colloid osmotic pressure. The colloid osmotic pressure of normal plasma is a weighted average reflecting the concentrations of albumin and globulin.

exert an osmotic pressure of approximately 1-2 mmHg. Changes in the protein concentration of the interstitial space are determined by (1) the volume of fluid in the interstitial space and (2) the rate at which protein is entering or leaving the space. If, for example, the capillaries become more permeable to protein (such as occurs during inflammation), plasma protein enters the interstitial space at an increased rate, and the interstitial protein concentration as well as interstitial colloid osmotic pressure increases.

Because capillary hydrostatic pressure is greater at the arterial end of the capillary, filtration is favored there; the lower capillary hydrostatic pressure at the venous end favors reabsorption. It is doubtful, however, that both filtration and reabsorption occur in every capillary. Instead, it appears that some capillaries exhibit filtration along most of their length and others exhibit reabsorption. On the average, however, capillaries act as would be predicted from the mean capillary hydrostatic pressure. For this reason, mean capillary hydrostatic pressure (P_c) is useful in predicting the result of various interventions on capillary fluid balance. If the representative numbers used above are considered, we get the following tally:

Forces favoring filtration out of capillaries:

capillary hydrostatic pressure: 18 mmHg
interstitial colloid osmotic pressure: 1 mmHg
total: 19 mmHg

Forces favoring reabsorption into capillaries:

interstitial hydrostatic pressure: − 7 mmHg
plasma colloid osmotic pressure: 25 mmHg
total: 18 mmHg

The forces favoring filtration essentially balance the forces favoring reabsorption. The slightly larger force favoring filtration, and the slight net filtration that occurs as a result, is balanced by the flow of lymph from the interstitial space. It is important to realize that the use of numbers here is only for the sake of illustration, and that any set of numbers is almost certainly in error. The point is that the colloid osmotic pressure difference between plasma and interstitial space of approximately 24 mmHg offsets almost perfectly the hydrostatic pressure difference between the plasma and the interstitial space. In addition, as will be stressed below, one should understand the ways in which each of the four forces can be altered to produce changes in plasma volume and in interstitial volume.

THE LYMPHATIC SYSTEM

The lymphatic system performs two important circulatory functions: (1) it returns proteins and excess interstitial fluid to the circulation, and (2) it serves as a pathway for the absorption of most lipids from the gastrointestinal tract. It will be the first of these functions that will concern us in this chapter. The lymphatic system consists of a network of extremely thin-walled vessels originating in the interstitial space throughout the body, coming together into larger vessels that generally accompany veins. Ultimately, the lymphatic drainage empties into the subclavian vein in the chest . At key confluence points, lymph nodes are present. Lymph is filtered through these nodes on its way to the subclavian vein.

Lymph is formed whenever the net forces favoring capillary filtration exceed the net forces favoring reabsorption. Flow of fluid from the lymphatic terminals to the subclavian vein occurs as a result of hydrostatic pressure differences between those two points. Because the subclavian vein pressure is low (similar to right atrial pressure), it is the pressure in the peripheral lymphatic vessels that determines the flow rate back to the circulation. The peripheral lymphatic pressure is influenced by the interstitial fluid hydrostatic pressure and the activity of the lymphatic pump. The interstitial hydrostatic pressure is determined by the volume of fluid in the interstitial space, as is shown in fig. 6-8. If the volume is increased, the interstitial pressure rises, as does lymphatic flow.

The lymphatic pump consists of the combination of valves in the lymphatic channels and various forces tending to compress the lymphatics. The valves are arranged so that any compression pushes lymph toward the chest. Various forces tending to compress the lymphatics are (1) muscle contractions, (2) arterial pulsations, and (3) all other forms of external compression. During exercise, for example, lymph flow from muscle increases threefold to fourfold because muscle contractions raise lymph pressure and force lymph toward the chest.

EDEMA

Edema can be defined as an abnormally high interstitial fluid volume. Edema is caused by (1) an upset in the hydrostatic or osmotic forces across the capillary such that filtration is favored or (2) obstructions that impair the return of lymph to the circulation. Several factors militate against the formation of edema, and these have been called the *"safety factors"* against edema. The first factor is reflected in the curve relating the interstitial fluid pressure to interstitial fluid volume (fig. 6-8). Since only very small increases in volume are necessary to cause marked increases in interstitial pressure in the normal volume range, a slight tendency for increased filtration is soon counterbalanced by a slight increase in interstitial fluid volume and a marked increase in interstitial fluid pressure. This same increased interstitial fluid pressure results in the second safety factor, which is increased lymph flow. The third safety factor is the washout of interstitial fluid protein, which occurs as lymph flow increases. Since the colloid osmotic pressure of the interstitial fluid tends to pull fluid into the interstitial space, lowering the concentration of protein in the interstitial fluid decreases the tendency for net filtration and edema formation. These safety factors mean that marked increases in capillary hydrostatic pressure or decreases in plasma colloid osmotic pressure must occur before edema formation begins.

The most important causes of edema are (1) elevation of capillary hydrostatic pressure, (2) decreased plasma colloid osmotic pressure, (3) increased capillary permeability, and (4) obstruction of the lymphatics.

Capillary hydrostatic pressure is usually elevated because of increased venous pressure. The simplest cases are those involving partial obstruction of venous outflow (due to venous thrombosis, compression of veins by tumor, etc.). In this situation the elevated venous resistance raises capillary hydrostatic pressure (as was depicted in fig. 6-7) which causes increased net filtration. If the elevation in net filtration is small, it may be balanced by increased tissue hydrostatic pressure and lymph flow as soon as interstitial fluid volume has increased slightly (fig. 6-8). If filtration is too great, the volume of the interstitial space increases to the point where further elevations in volume produce only slight increases in interstitial pressure, and a balance may not be reached until a considerable increase in interstitial fluid volume (with clinically apparent edema) has occurred.

Plasma colloid osmotic pressure decreases (e.g., in patients with nephrotic syndrome) when plasma protein is lost through the kidneys (fig. 6-10). Minimal edema occurs until the colloid osmotic pressure is reduced 10-15 mmHg because of the safety factors discussed above. As the protein concentration falls, the plasma colloid pressure (tending to hold fluid in the capillaries) decreases, and fluid filters into the interstitial space. The interstitial space pressure rises as the interstitial fluid volume increases. The increased interstitial pressure acts directly against further filtration and also raises lymph flow, which slows the rise in interstitial fluid volume. When plasma colloid osmotic pressure falls by 10-15 mmHg, the safety factors are overwhelmed and edema is formed.

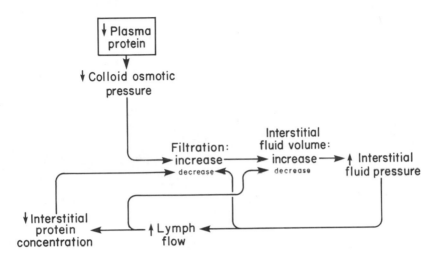

FIGURE 6-10.
Effect of decreased plasma protein concentration on interstitial fluid volume and pressure, lymph flow, and transcapillary filtration.

The inflammatory response, which will be discussed in the section on cutaneous circulation in chapter 7, causes arteriolar dilation and increased vascular permeability to protein (fig. 6-11). Arteriolar vasodilation results in elevated vascular hydrostatic pressure (fig. 6-7), and the increased vascular permeability to protein raises interstitial protein concentration and interstitial colloid osmotic pressure. Thus two forces operate to increase filtration in the edema associated with inflammation.

If lymphatic channels are obstructed due to infection, surgical removal or irradiation of lymph nodes, interstitial protein cannot be removed from the interstitial space (fig. 6-12). The elevated interstitial space pressure might allow water and electrolytes to be reabsorbed, but the concentration gradient for protein means that it cannot be returned to the capillaries directly. As protein accumulates (and eventually reaches the capillary concentration) the colloid osmotic pressure difference can no longer balance the capillary hydrostatic pressure difference, and gross edema results.

Edema in the lungs *(pulmonary edema)* has especially devastating consequences. As the exceedingly small distance between

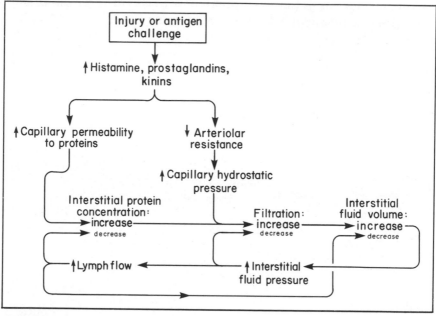

FIGURE 6-11.
Events in the inflammatory response.

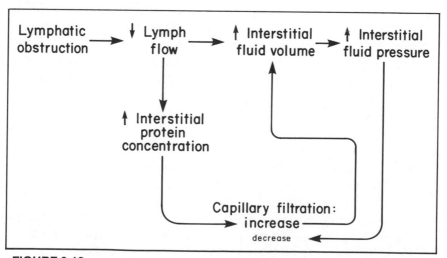

FIGURE 6-12.
Effect of lymphatic obstruction on edema formation.

the blood cells and the alveolar gas is increased by edema fluid, gas exchange is diminished and the patient begins to drown in his or her own fluid. The lungs are kept dry by the same factors that operate in other tissues, but with important differences. The pulmonary capillary pressure is only 8-10 mmHg, and interstitial colloid osmotic pressure is very high, approximately 14 mmHg. When microvascular pressure is increased, for example, in left heart failure, four safety factors prevent the buildup of fluid in the alveoli. The most significant of these is lymph flow, which normally carries off excess filtration. Second, the capillary endothelium has a very low K_F, so the rate of filtration in response to a given pressure difference is small. Third, the microvascular barrier to plasma protein is very tight. This means that the increased lymph flow associated with filtration quickly washes out interstitial protein and lowers interstitial fluid colloid osmotic pressure, which raises the colloid osmotic pressure gradient and reduces filtration. Finally, the alveolar epithelial lining is highly impermeable to any edema fluid that accumulates in the interstitial space. This means that the fluid is directed into the lymphatics rather than flooding the alveoli. The net effect of these safety factors is that left atrial pressure must increase to 20-25 mmHg before pulmonary edema may occur.

Suggested Readings

Bohr DF, Somlyo AP, Sparks HV Jr. (eds.): *Handbook of Physiology. Section 2: The Cardiovascular System.* Bethesda, American Physiological Society, vol. 2, 1980

Guyton AC: *Textbook of Medical Physiology.* 6th ed. Philadelphia, W. B. Saunders Co., 1981, pp 358-380

Johnson PC: Principles of peripheral circulatory control. In *Peripheral Circulation.* Edited by PC Johnson. New York, John Wiley and Sons, 1978

Landis EM: The capillary circulation. In *Circulation of the Blood: Men and Ideas.* Edited by AP Fishman and DW Richards. Bethesda, American Physiological Society, 1982, pp 355-406

Staub NC, Taylor AE (eds.): *Edema.* New York, Raven Press, 1984

Chapter 7

Regulation of Blood Flow

This chapter describes the factors controlling the flow of blood through the various organs of the body. Organ blood flow is determined by the pressure drop across the organ and the resistance to blood flow offered by the vessels within it. All of the organs to be discussed, except the lungs and liver, are in parallel (see chapter 1) and are exposed to the same arterial pressure. In most situations the mean arterial pressure is held relatively constant by the neurogenic and humoral mechanisms discussed in chapter 5. Variations in organ blood flow are caused by changes in vascular resistance, that is, vasodilation and vasoconstriction. Vascular resistance can be altered not only by neural and humoral mechanisms, but also by local mechanisms within the organ. Resistance changes caused by neural and/or humoral factors usually subserve homeostatic mechanisms of importance to the whole body; for example, regulation of mean arterial pressure or body temperature. In addition to these remote controllers of vascular resistance, each organ has a set of local control mechanisms that best serve its function. For example, skeletal muscle has powerful local mechanisms that adjust flow to meet its increased metabolic needs during exercise. Skin, on the other hand,[1] has an elaborate local vascular control system that responds to injury. A combination of local and remote regulatory mechanisms determines the vascular resistance of a given organ at any one time.

THE PULMONARY CIRCULATION

One of the two major exceptions to the parallel arrangement of the vasculature is the pulmonary circulation. The entire cardiac output

---

[1] Or any place else, for that matter.

flows from the right heart through the pulmonary circulation. The major function of the lungs is to provide a surface for the exchange of gases between blood and alveoli. To accomplish this, blood is passed through a low-resistance network of pulmonary capillaries. The capillaries are separated from the alveolar gas by a thin alveolar membrane, across which the exchange of gases can easily occur. The total alveolar surface area available for exchange is approximately 100 m².

Pulmonary arterial pulse pressure (fig. 7-1) is determined by right heart stroke volume and pulmonary arterial compliance. Mean

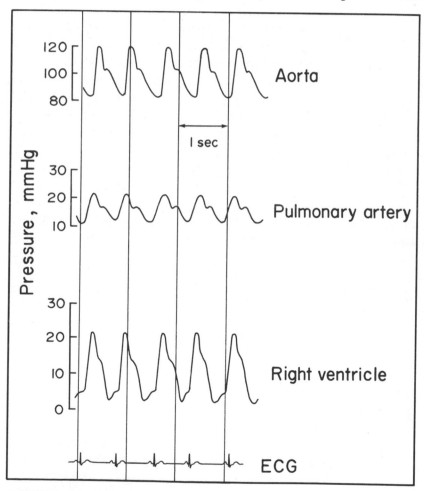

FIGURE 7-1.
Pressure tracing against time for the aorta, pulmonary artery, and right ventricle.

pulmonary arterial pressure is influenced by cardiac output and total pulmonary vascular resistance, and is 13 mmHg, with a systolic
pressure of 22 and a diastolic pressure of 8 mmHg. Left atrial pressure is approximately 5 mmHg, and thus the mean pressure drop
across the entire pulmonary circuit is roughly 8 mmHg. The vascular resistance of the pulmonary bed with a cardiac output of 5.5 L/
min is:

$$R_{pulmonary} = P/F = 8/5.5 = 1.4 \, mmHg \times min/L$$

as compared with the total peripheral resistance of the systemic circuit:

$$TPR = MAP/CO = 93/5.5 = 17 \, mmHg \times min/L$$

The exceedingly low pulmonary vascular resistance reflects the relatively large vessel radius on both the arterial and the venous sides
of the pulmonary circulation. The pulmonary pulse pressure is also
lower than systemic pulse pressure (14 in contrast to 40 mmHg) because compliance of pulmonary arteries is much lower than that of
the aorta and large systemic arteries.

When cardiac output increases, as with exercise, flow through
the lungs must increase also. One might expect pulmonary arterial
pressure to rise dramatically as the right heart forces increasingly
more blood flow through the lungs. However, very small changes in
pulmonary arterial pressure occur with threefold to fourfold
changes in cardiac output because small increases in pulmonary arterial pressure enlarge the highly compliant pulmonary arteries and
veins enough to decrease pulmonary vascular resistance dramatically. In fact, a 5 mmHg increase in pulmonary arterial pressure resulting from increased cardiac output causes pulmonary resistance
to decrease by a factor of four.

Perfusion of the lungs in an upright person is not uniform because the vascular transmural pressure is greater at the base than at
the apex of the lungs. One component of transmural pressure, the
pressure on the outside of the alveolar capillaries, is the same as alveolar air: on the average, atmospheric pressure. The pressure within
alveolar capillaries is much higher at the base than at the apex of the
lungs because of the hydrostatic column of blood between these
two areas. Pressure in the alveolar capillaries at the apex is less than
the alveolar pressure during at least part of expiration. When alveolar pressure is highest the vessels collapse, raising resistance to

flow. Distention of vessels in the base of the lungs by the higher hydrostatic transmural pressure lowers the resistance of vessels in this area. Thus, when a person is upright, blood flow through the base of the lungs is much higher than blood flow through apical areas (fig. 7-2).

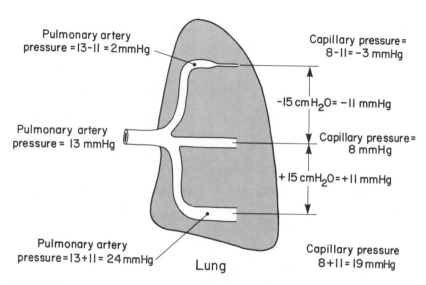

FIGURE 7-2.

Effects of hydrostatic gradients in the lungs of an upright individual. In an upright individual the mean pulmonary arterial pressure is 13 mmHg, and capillary pressure is 8 mmHg. The hydrostatic force on the blood in the lungs raises these pressures to 24 and 19 mmHg (respectively) at the base, and lowers them to 2 and −3 mmHg at the apex of the lungs. The higher transmural pressure at the base of the lungs distends the vessels and lowers local vascular resistance to flow. The lower transmural pressure at the apex causes vessels to collapse, which raises resistance to flow, especially during expiration when alveolar pressure is highest and transmural pressure is lowest. These events explain the gradient of blood flow from the base (where it is highest) to the apex (where it is lowest).

Respiratory movements have a profound effect on pulmonary blood volume. Resting pulmonary blood volume is approximately 600 mL. With a deep inspiration it increases to 1000 mL, and with full expiration it decreases to 200 mL. These changes in vascular volume occur because expansion and contraction of the chest alter the pressure on the outside of the pulmonary vessels. The use of positive pressure ventilation causes decreased transmural pressure, just as occurs during expiration; it tends to collapse pulmonary vessels, lowering pulmonary vascular volume and raising pulmonary vascular resistance. The rise in pulmonary vascular resistance can be great enough to impede the output of the right heart, thereby decreasing left ventricular filling and left cardiac output.

With a resting cardiac output, red blood cells spend approximately 0.75 sec in the pulmonary capillaries; this time is reduced to 0.33 sec during exercise when cardiac output is much higher. With a high cardiac output, the shorter pulmonary transit time is just adequate to allow the pO_2 of the capillary blood to reach the pO_2 of normal alveolar gas. If alveolar pO_2 is lowered significantly by exposure to high altitude or by disease, there may be insufficient time for complete oxygenation of hemoglobin during exercise. This results in a marked reduction in exercise capacity.

The vascular smooth muscle of the pulmonary arteries and arterioles is scanty, and that of the veins is almost nonexistent. The lack of smooth muscle explains the thin walls and large compliances of these vessels. In general, it also means that active vascular responses in this bed are relatively weak. The exception to this is one important local control mechanism: pulmonary arterioles constrict in response to lowered alveolar pO_2. If a portion of lung does not receive adequate ventilation (e.g., because of a blocked airway), pO_2 decreases in the alveolar gas. The decrease in alveolar pO_2 results in pulmonary arteriolar vasoconstriction and reduces blood flow to that area. That portion of the cardiac output is then shunted to another area of the lungs where oxygenation can occur. Fortunately, diminished pulmonary arterial pO_2, as occurs in exercise, does not cause constriction of pulmonary arterioles.

Table 7-1. Metabolic Functions of Pulmonary Endothelium

Metabolic Process	Mechanism
Conversion of angiotensin I to angiotensin II	Converting enzyme; a carboxypeptidase located on the luminal surface of endothelial cells
Serotonin, norepinephrine, and epinephrine uptake	Uptake by carrier(s) and oxidation by monoamine oxidase
Bradykinin inactivation	Hydrolysis by converting enzyme
Adenine nucleotide removal	Dephosphorylation by phosphatases on luminal surface; uptake of adenosine
Prostaglandin removal	Uptake and oxidation
Prostaglandin (especially PGI_2) synthesis	Arachidonic acid cascade in endothelial cells

The pulmonary microcirculation performs a second very important service, the *metabolic function of the lung.* Pulmonary endothelial cells are capable of metabolizing a wide variety of substances presented to them from the systemic circulation. Some of these are shown in table 7-1, along with the mechanisms responsible for their metabolism. This function may be important for survival when injured tissues such as skeletal muscle release large amounts of vasoactive substances, for example, adenine nucleotides and prostaglandins. Perhaps the best understood metabolic function of the lung is the conversion of the inactive decapeptide *angiotensin I* to the active octapeptide *angiotensin II* (table 7-1).

SKELETAL MUSCLE BLOOD FLOW

Skeletal muscle blood flow changes over a wide range, and because skeletal muscle constitutes 40-50% of the body weight, changes in the blood flow of this tissue require large changes in cardiac output. During exercise, flow through red, high-oxidative muscle is higher than flow through white, low-oxidative fibers.[2] The information presented here is representative of mixed skeletal muscle containing both extremes as well as intermediate fiber types.

Figure 7-3 illustrates the 150-fold range over which skeletal muscle flow can vary (with arterial pressure constant at 93 mmHg). Resting blood flow is approximately 2-3 mL/100 g of muscle/min, or a total of 1 L/min for a 70 kg person. When sympathetic vasoconstrictor nerves are maximally stimulated, blood flow falls to 20% of its resting value. During vigorous exercise, muscle blood flow may increase to 80-100 mL/100 g/min.

At rest, arterioles of skeletal muscle exhibit substantial contractile tone. This is evidenced by the 40-fold increase in blood flow that occurs with exercise. The part of the resting arteriolar tone caused by sympathetic vasoconstrictor nerves can be determined by observing how much blood flow increases when the nerves are cut. When the experiment is done, blood flow increases to 6-9 mL/100 g/min. The portion of the arteriolar tone caused by nerves is

---

[2]Skeletal muscles from various sites exhibit a wide range of maximum oxygen consumption (low- versus high-oxidation fibers). In general, high-oxidative fibers contain more myoglobulin (and are red) than do low-oxidative fibers (which are white). High- and low-oxidative fiber types are often mixed within the same muscle.

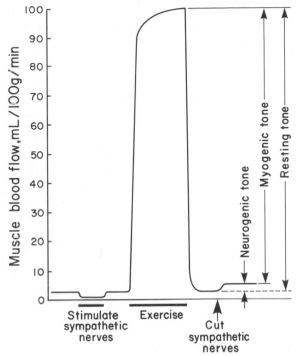

FIGURE 7-3.
Changes in skeletal muscle blood flow associated with stimulation of sympathetic nerves, exercise, and cutting of sympathetic nerves.

called *neurogenic tone.* Figure 7-3 shows that neurogenic tone accounts for only a small portion of resting arteriolar tone. The portion of resting arteriolar smooth muscle tone not caused by nerves is referred to as *myogenic tone,* indicating that it originates in the smooth muscle. Most vascular smooth muscle exhibits tone, but the relative amounts of myogenic, humoral, and neurogenic tone of arterioles varies a great deal from organ to organ.

The tremendous increase in skeletal muscle blood flow with exercise, called *exercise hyperemia,* is caused by a variety of local vasodilator mechanisms (see figure 6-5). These mechanisms can overwhelm whatever sympathetic and myogenic tones are present and elicit maximum vasodilation. The local metabolic vasodilators include K^+, which is released with skeletal muscle action potentials and accumulates in the interstitial space. In addition, muscle contraction results in an increase in the number of osmotically active particles within the skeletal muscle cells. Water moves into the cells, raising the interstitial osmolarity; increased osmolarity also causes vasodilation. With intense exercise, lowered tissue pO_2 may lower the vessel wall pO_2 and result in vasodilation. Other factors, for example, adenosine, prostaglandins, and increased H^+ concentration may play a role in causing exercise hyperemia.

Neurogenic vasoconstriction resulting from baroreceptor or chemoreceptor reflexes occurs in resting skeletal muscle. This is the result of norepinephrine binding to α-adrenergic receptors. Sympathetic stimulation in the presence of exercise causes very little decrease in flow. This is because K^+, increased osmolarity, prostaglandins, and adenosine not only relax vascular smooth muscle, they also inhibit release of norepinephrine from sympathetic nerve varicosities.

Stimulation of sympathetic cholinergic fibers to skeletal muscle results in vasodilation via muscarinic cholinergic receptors. The increased blood flow resulting from activation of these neurons occurs in *anticipation* of exercise, but does not contribute significantly to the maintenance of increased blood flow during exercise.

Increased circulating epinephrine from the adrenal medulla also contributes to the increased blood flow during exercise by binding to vascular smooth muscle β-adrenergic receptors.

Within limits, if mean arterial pressure to skeletal muscle is changed, flow is held relatively constant by adjustment of vascular resistance, again by local mechanisms. This is called *autoregulation of blood flow.* Two general mechanisms are at work. (1) *Metabolic autoregulation:* when pressure is increased, the increased flow washes out vasodilatory substances, perhaps some of the same ones involved in exercise hyperemia. As the dilators are washed out, vasoconstriction results, which tends to return flow toward the control level. (2) *Myogenic autoregulation:* when pressure is increased, the walls of arterioles are stretched. The vascular smooth muscle responds to stretch by contracting. The resulting contraction brings flow back toward the control level. Both of these mechanisms also work in the opposite direction, that is, with decreased arterial pressure, vasodilation results. Autoregulation of blood flow may have important systemic hemodynamic consequences in the long-term regulation of cardiac output and mean arterial pressure (chapter 8).

If the blood supply to skeletal muscle is stopped for a time, a period of increased flow follows the release of the occlusion. This is called *reactive hyperemia,* and it is also caused by the combination of a myogenic response and accumulation of vasodilator metabolites.

The volume of blood in resting muscle is approximately 850 mL, or 15% of the total blood volume. Roughly 75% of this is in veins. Because the veins of skeletal muscle are poorly innervated, only 100-200 mL of this blood can be moved to the central blood volume by sympathetic venoconstriction. This is not a hemodynamically significant volume under most conditions. Much more volume can be moved by the *muscle pump*. In the extremities, veins of subcutaneous tissue and muscle are equipped with valves. When the veins are compressed by the enlarged bellies of contracting skeletal muscle, blood is moved toward the heart. This process is described in detail in chapter 8.

CUTANEOUS BLOOD FLOW

Skin is subjected to wider swings in temperature and more trauma than any other organ. Skin is also the site of heat loss from the body. Heat is conducted poorly through the fatty subcutaneous layer; therefore blood flow brings most excess heat to the skin. In normal individuals, blood flow is seldom so low that adequate nutrition of skin becomes a factor influencing skin blood flow. In light of these facts, it is not surprising that the control of skin blood flow is mainly related to the response to injury and the regulation of body temperature.

An unusual aspect of the cutaneous circulation is the rich venous plexus, which provides a huge surface area for heat loss. This venous plexus is also responsible for the red-to-blue hue of skin that is superimposed on skin color in all but the most highly pigmented individuals. If this subcutaneous plexus is dilated, the color of blood, whether red, blue, or intermediate, markedly affects skin color. If the venous plexus is constricted, the color of the skin is mainly determined by skin pigmentation. The skin color due to the blood in the venous plexus is an important indicator of skin blood flow and oxygenation. Intense red hues indicate high blood flow, far in excess of oxygen needs of the tissue. With partial venous occlusion, the flow is low and the vessels dilate because of local metabolite accumulation. As a result of the low flow, a great deal of oxygen is extracted and the skin has an intense bluish hue *(cyanosis)*. When low blood flow is caused by arterial occlusion or vasoconstriction, the venous plexus contains little blood and a cadaveric pallor results.

Arteriovenous anastomoses occur in the skin of the hands, feet, and ears. These are large-bore channels, with a thick smooth muscle coat, that allow blood to go directly from arterioles to the venous plexus. Their large radii permit an extremely high flow that does not supply nutrients to skin (because capillaries are bypassed), but allows heat loss from the venous plexus.

Skin blood flow can vary from 400 mL/min, when a 70 kg person is at rest in a thermally neutral environment, to 3.5 L/min with elevated body temperature in a very hot environment.

Both arteries and veins of skin are heavily innervated by sympathetic nerve fibers and respond to norepinephrine release by α-adrenergic receptor-mediated constriction.

Skin blood flow is affected by changes in local skin temperature and by changes in hypothalamic or core temperature. For example, hand skin blood flow increases with local skin temperature when the hand is immersed in water of various temperatures between 10° C and 45° C (fig. 7-4). If the ambient temperature for the person is so high that cutaneous vasodilation is necessary to dissipate (core) heat, flow will be higher at a given water temperature. If the ambient temperature is low, flow in the hand will be lower at a given water temperature. The increase in blood flow resulting from the rise in local temperature is caused partly by a reflex decrease in sympathetic vasoconstrictor tone and partly by a decreased sensitivity of the vascular smooth muscle to norepinephrine. If the local skin temperature is below 10° C, cold vasodilation occurs. Cold vasodilation results from a direct effect of cold on the vascular smooth muscle, producing relaxation. Cold vasodilation usually alternates with periods of vasoconstriction. Pain resulting from exposure to cold occurs simultaneously with vasodilation. The periods of increased blood flow may save the skin from damage caused by freezing, with the alternate periods of vasoconstriction favoring retention of body heat. When the local skin temperature is above 45° C the result is burn injury, which will be described below; blood flow is very high in this situation.

The effects of body temperature on skin blood flow are initiated by changes in hypothalamic temperature, which result in changes in (1) sympathetic neural activity, (2) sweat gland activity and the re-

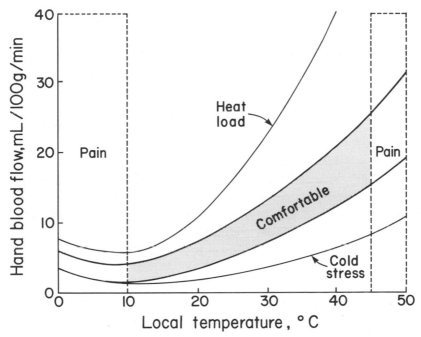

FIGURE 7-4.
Effect of temperature on hand blood flow. Changes in hand blood flow occur with changes in local hand temperature caused by immersing hand in water of various temperatures. Hand blood flow increases much more with increased local temperature if the whole body is exposed to a heat load (e.g., a hot room). Cold stress keeps hand blood flow low despite local warming. If the general environment is comfortable, the results are in between.

lease of bradykinin, and (3) possibly another direct neurogenic vasodilator system. When ambient temperature is low and the hypothalamic temperature falls, cutaneous blood flow can be less than 1 mL/100 g/min. As ambient temperature increases, so does skin blood flow. First the arteriovenous anastomoses open, and then regular artery-capillary-venous circuits become dilated. Opening of the arteriovenous anastomoses results from the removal of sympathetic constrictor activity. Vasodilation of the rest of the skin blood vessels proceeds by the same mechanism until all sympathetic constrictor tone is withdrawn. At that point skin blood flow is approximately 25-30 mL/100 g/min. Further increases in skin blood flow are associated with sweating, which occurs at high hypothalamic temperatures. Increased sweat gland activity is accompanied by the release of a powerful vasodilator called *bradykinin.* This polypeptide causes further increases in skin blood flow to as much as 100-150 mL/100 g/min. There is considerable debate over whether these two mechanisms adequately explain the increase in skin blood flow that occurs with increased hypothalamic temperature. There may be another vasodilator system, for example, one involving release of histamine.

When blood pressure and temperature regulation compete, temperature regulation predominates. For example, when a soldier stands at attention in the hot sun, skin blood flow and venous volume are elevated because of the hypothalamic response to increased heat load. This response predominates over the tendency of the baroreceptor reflex to lower skin blood flow and volume (see chapter 5). The cutaneous vasodilation in response to heat load results in a lower total peripheral resistance as well as displacement of blood from the central blood volume to the veins of the skin. In this situation arterial pressure may fall low enough to result in loss of consciousness.

Another example of the competition between thermoregulation and blood pressure regulation is vigorous exercise in a hot environment. During such exercise, 3-4 L/min of cardiac output may flow through the skin. Because this blood is unavailable for exercising skeletal muscle, muscular performance is limited by thermal regulatory demand. Finally, if a patient with hypotension (caused by loss of blood) is warmed too much, increased skin blood flow and venous volume can compromise central blood volume and reduce cardiac output. In summary, thermal regulation frequently dominates blood pressure regulation when a conflict develops. The dominance of temperature over blood pressure regulation probably occurs within the central nervous system.

The *triple response* (fig. 7-5) is observed following many types of skin injury, including mechanical and thermal damage and allergic reactions. With mechanical injuries, such as a scrape caused by a sharp object, three events usually occur. First, a *red line* develops directly under the area of the injury, reflecting local vasodilation resulting from histamine and prostaglandin release. Second, a *flare* of redness appears around the injured area as a result of the "axon reflex." Pain fiber action potentials are propagated toward the central nervous system, but return (without leaving skin) by way of special nerve branches to arterioles in the area. A vasodilator (perhaps ATP or substance P) is released and results in the red flare surrounding the injury. The third component of the triple response is the formation of a *wheal.* A wheal is a local area of cutaneous edema caused by increased capillary hydrostatic pressure and permeability to

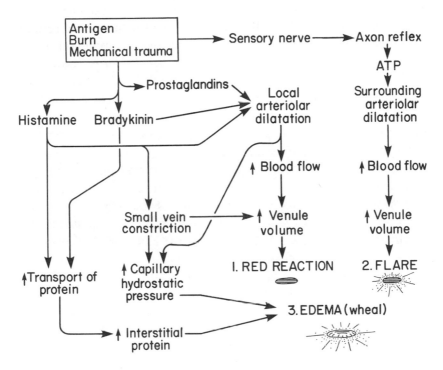

FIGURE 7-5.
Response of blood flow in skin to injury.

protein (see chapter 6) produced as a consequence of histamine, prostaglandin, and bradykinin release. Similar events occur with damage caused by thermal injury or allergic reactions.

If sufficient pressure is applied to the skin, blood flow can be stopped. When the pressure is removed by, for example, the person's changing his or her position, reactive hyperemia (indicated by an area of redness) develops. Reactive hyperemia is caused by either a local accumulation of vasodilator metabolites or a myogenic response, as in skeletal muscle.

CEREBRAL BLOOD FLOW

Brain blood flow is almost 15% of cardiac output, and brain oxygen consumption is 20% of resting oxygen consumption. Thus a tissue constituting 2% of the body weight demands a significant fraction of both the transported oxygen and cardiac output at rest. Diminished cerebral blood flow and oxygen supply quickly result in loss of consciousness. In general, loss of consciousness is the most maladaptive event possible, and it should not be surprising that cerebral blood flow is usually held constant. Autoregulation is the most significant mechanism responsible for regulation of cerebral blood flow. Decreased mean arterial pressure does not result in a proportional fall in cerebral blood flow unless the pressure drops below 60 mmHg. The cerebral arteriolar dilation that holds flow relatively constant under these circumstances is due to rising tissue pCO_2 (and H^+ concentration), falling pO_2, a myogenic response, and increased interstitial adenosine concentration. Increased metabolism associated with brain cell activity results in increased blood flow, oxygen consumption, and glucose uptake. The increased blood flow is mediated by changes in tissue pCO_2 (and H^+), pO_2, K^+, and adenosine.

Increased arterial blood pCO_2 and decreased arterial blood pO_2 cause dramatic increases in cerebral blood flow. Arterial CO_2 increases blood flow by elevating interstitial H^+ concentration, which dilates arterioles. Decreased arterial pO_2 causes vasodilation by its direct effect on vascular smooth muscle and by increasing adenosine production.

Under most conditions autonomic neural activity does not interfere with these local responses, all of which appear to have adaptive value in holding the environment of the brain as constant as possible. In this context the baroreceptor response can be looked upon as a reflex designed to maintain the perfusion pressure of the brain. However, there is now evidence that sympathetic neural activity can modify both autoregulatory responses and the response of cerebral arterioles to pCO_2 (H^+) and pO_2. We do not know whether neural mechanisms play a physiologically significant role in the regulation of cerebral blood flow, or whether in some cases they could account for pathophysiological events such as spasm of cerebral arteries.

Elevated intracranial pressure raises mean arterial pressure by directly stimulating the medullary cardiovascular center, which causes an increase in total peripheral resistance. This is called the *Cushing reflex*. The adaptive value of this reflex is interesting. Since the cranium is a rigid container, rising intracranial pressure would cause increased pressure on the outside of the blood vessels of the brain, tending to collapse them. An increase in mean arterial pressure tends to prevent collapse of blood vessels and to maintain blood flow in spite of the rising intracranial pressure. The increased pressure invokes the baroreceptor response, which slows heart rate. The net effect is an increase in mean arterial pressure despite the reflex slowing of heart rate.

SPLANCHNIC BLOOD FLOW

Splanchnic blood flow is defined as flow to the stomach, spleen, intestines, pancreas, and liver. Blood flow to these organs is supplied by three major branches of the aorta. In addition to its arterial blood supply, the liver receives venous drainage from the stomach, spleen, intestine, and pancreas *(hepatic portal system)*. Seventy percent of liver blood flow is from the portal system and 30% is from the hepatic artery.

Ingestion of food results in increased blood flow to each organ as it becomes involved in the digestive and absorptive processes. Active secretory tissues like the gastric mucosa, pancreas, liver, and small intestinal mucosa need large increases in flow to supply the large volumes of secretions they produce, that is, approximately 2 L during an average meal. In addition, the secretory activity and increased motility of the gut smooth muscle require an increased supply of oxygen. The mechanisms causing the increased blood flow include bradykinin release from endocrine glands (analogous to that described with reference to the sweat gland). There is also release of vasodilator metabolites as in skeletal muscle. Finally, 5-hydroxytryptamine is released from enterochromaffin cells during digestion, and this causes increased intestinal blood flow.

Splanchnic blood vessels are richly innervated by sympathetic fibers and respond to increased sympathetic neural activity with vasoconstriction mediated by α-receptors. This is very important for maintenance of blood pressure and central blood volume because the splanchnic circulation receives 1.5 L/min in a 70 kg person (25% of the resting cardiac output). This flow can be diverted to more vital areas when needed. In addition, the splanchnic circulation acts as a volume reservoir containing between 1 and 1.5 L of blood; approximately 40-50% of this can be transferred to the central blood volume via venoconstriction. Splanchnic vasoconstriction occurs with activation of the baroreceptor and chemoreceptor reflexes and the defense response. Increased hypothalamic temperature causes sympathetic splanchnic vasoconstriction, which compliments the cutaneous vasodilation. Thus there is a redistribution of both cardiac output and blood volume from the splanchnic to the cutaneous circulation. Splanchnic vasoconstriction also occurs with exercise. This causes cardiac output to be shifted away from the gut to skeletal muscle and helps maintain central blood volume. This is especially important during exercise in a warm environment when both muscle and skin blood flow must increase.

RENAL BLOOD FLOW

The kidneys receive approximately 1200 mL of blood per minute, or 20% of the cardiac output. The kidney vasculature is richly supplied with sympathetic nerves, and increasing sympathetic neural activity leads to α-receptor-mediated vasoconstriction and increased vascular resistance to flow. As in the case of the splanchnic circulation, a variety of situations including baroreceptor reflex activation (e.g., during orthostasis) and the defense response result in renal vasoconstriction. Activation of sympathetic nerves to kidney arterioles often results in only a modest decrease in renal blood flow, but this decrease amplifies the direct effect of sympathetic nerves on the release of renin via the β-receptor as described in chapter 5. In addition, the glomerular filtration rate tends to fall with decreased renal blood flow. This means that renal vasoconstriction reduces the filtration of Na^+. Thus even small changes in renal blood flow may have very important effects on the control of blood volume. The cortical areas of the kidney where juxtaglomerular cells are located are more affected by sympathetic nerve stimulation than are medullary areas.

Changes in mean arterial pressure produce very small changes in renal blood flow over a considerable range of pressures (fig. 7-6). This autoregulation of blood flow is caused by resistance vessel constriction associated with increased arterial pressure. The mechanism for this increased resistance involves (1) vasoconstriction (directly in response to increased transmural pressure, i.e., the myogenic response) and/or (2) the renin-angiotensin system.

The relationship between renal blood flow and metabolism is unusual. First, because of the extremely high blood flow of the kidneys, only 5-10% of the available oxygen in arterial blood flow is extracted (by contrast, resting skeletal muscle extracts 50-60% of the available oxygen). When flow to the kidney is decreased, metabolism slows because there is less glomerular filtration and less energy-requiring tubular transport. Thus in the kidney, flow determines metabolism, whereas in most organs metabolism determines flow.

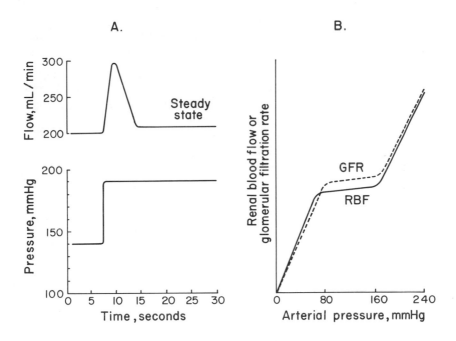

FIGURE 7-6.
Autoregulation of renal blood flow (RBF) with changes in arterial pressure. Panel A shows the renal blood flow response to a sudden elevation in pressure. Flow increases and then rapidly returns toward the control level. Panel B shows the steady-state values for a variety of pressures. Note the small change in RBF associated with changes in arterial pressure between 80 and 160 mmHg. Glomerular filtration rate (GFR) shows a similiar plateau.

CORONARY BLOOD FLOW

Coronary blood flow is determined by four factors: (1) the pressure driving flow through the coronary bed, (2) the compression of the coronary vessels caused by ventricular contraction, (3) the metabolic activity of the myocardium, and (4) the activity of the coronary nerves. Coronary blood flow in a 70 kg person ranges from approximately 200 mL/min at rest to approximately 1050 mL/min with maximum vasodilation, for example, with exercise.

Blood flow through the myocardium is determined by the pressure difference between the inflow and outflow points, as is true for flow through any organ. The coronary bed represents a special case, however, because the heart produces its own pressure gradient. If for some reason the heart fails to maintain the mean arterial pressure, coronary blood flow tends to fall, depriving the heart of oxygen and further depressing its ability to pump blood and maintain arterial pressure. This vicious cycle is unique to the heart.

During systole the compressive force of the ventricular contraction greatly reduces coronary blood flow. Figure 7-7 shows that most left ventricular coronary blood flow occurs during diastole.[3]

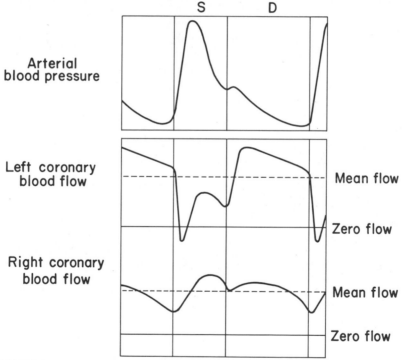

FIGURE 7-7.
Right and left coronary blood flow throughout the cardiac cycle. During systole (S) left coronary flow decreases due to compression of the coronary vessels by ventricular muscle. During diastole (D) left coronary flow increases as the ventricle relaxes, and then declines with the fall in diastolic pressure. Changes in right coronary blood flow (supplying chiefly the right ventricle) are much smaller because the compressive forces offered by the right ventricular muscle are less.

[3]In this context, you might wish to ponder the survival value of a relatively high diastolic pressure. With aortic insufficiency, the lowered diastolic pressure leads to poor perfusion of the myocardium.

During systole, flow virtually stops in the subendocardium because the transmural vessels are compressed (fig. 7-8). During the period of systolic compression, when flow is slowed or stopped, oxygen is supplied by *myoglobin* present in heart muscle. This protein binds oxygen and releases it at low pO_2's. During diastole, flow to the

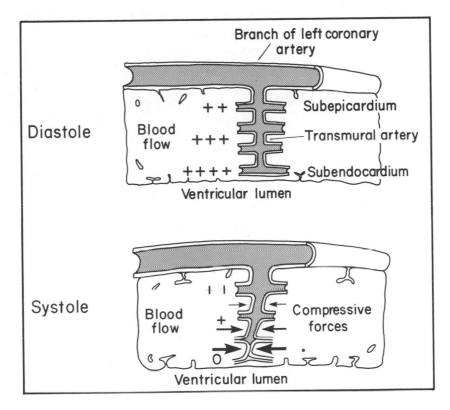

FIGURE 7-8.
Effect of compression on ventricular blood flow. During diastole left ventricular blood flow is highest in the subendocardium (+ + + +) and lowest in the subepicardium(+ +). During systole compressive forces associated with contraction of the myocardium collapse transmural arteries and flow to the subendocardium stops (0).

subendocardium increases dramatically, making up for the cessation of flow during systole. As heart rate increases and the duration of diastole decreases, there is less and less time for subendocardial flow. A normal individual has enough vasodilator capacity in reserve[4] so that metabolically induced vasodilation more than com-

[4]This is known as the *coronary reserve,* which is defined as the additional vasodilator capacity present under a particular set of conditions.

pensates for the decrease in duration of subendocardial flow. With partial coronary artery obstruction the coronary autoregulatory reserve in the endocardium can become exhausted, and inadequate blood may be supplied to the subendocardial myocardium during diastole. This is responsible for the high prevalence of subendocardial myocardial infarctions.

The most significant influence on coronary blood flow is myocardial metabolism. Whenever the use of ATP increases, oxygen consumption also increases because over 95% of ATP synthesis by the heart is aerobic. Under basal conditions 60% of arterial oxygen is extracted from the blood as it passes through coronary capillaries. If increased oxygen consumption occurs because of increased ATP use associated with increased heart rate and/or force development, little additional oxygen can be extracted from blood. For this reason, the required increase in oxygen must be supplied by increasing blood flow. The increased blood flow results from arteriolar dilation in response to local vasodilator metabolites. The metabolites thought to be most important are adenosine and K^+.

Coronary vascular smooth muscle contains α- and β-adrenergic, as well as muscarinic cholinergic, receptors. Norepinephrine released from nerve endings binds to α-adrenergic receptors, which is a stimulus for vasoconstriction. This stimulus is normally overwhelmed by the metabolic vasodilation resulting from increased myocardial metabolism. Increased sympathetic nervous system activity to coronary vessels does not occur without a coinciding increase in neural activity to the myocardium. Because the metabolic vasodilators mentioned above compete successfully with α-adrenergic vasoconstriction, the direct vasoconstrictor effects of sympathetic stimulation on coronary blood flow are usually hidden. For example, increased sympathetic neural activity to the heart in response to activation of the baroreceptor reflex raises oxygen consumption and causes metabolic vasodilation. Simultaneously, there is increased binding of norepinephrine to coronary α-adrenergic receptors. The resulting vasodilation is only slightly less than would occur in the absence of the coinciding α-stimulation. However, it is possible that neural vasoconstrictor influences could be much more important in individuals with coronary artery disease.[5]

---

[5]The idea that myocardial ischemia is linked to the emotions has been with us a long time. After experiencing repeated attacks of chest pain during periods of excitement or anger, John Hunter, the great 18th-century anatomist, predicted that his "life was in the hands of any rascal who chose to annoy and tease" him. He proved correct, dying shortly after a heated argument at a meeting of the board of governors of St. George's Hospital.

Stimulation of parasympathetic nerves to the heart results in increased binding of acetylcholine to coronary muscarinic cholinergic receptors. Because the concurrent decrease in heart rate reduces metabolic vasodilation, there is competition between a direct neural influence on the coronary arterial system and an indirect influence via myocardial metabolism. As is the case with sympathetic stimulation, metabolism predominates and the net effect of parasympathetic stimulation is reduced coronary blood flow.

Suggested Readings

Berne RM, Levy MN (eds.): *Cardiovascular Physiology.* 4th ed. St. Louis, The C. V. Mosby Company, 1981, pp 223-252

Johnson PC (ed.): *Peripheral Circulation.* New York, John Wiley and Sons, 1978

Shepherd JT, Vanhoutte PM: *The Human Cardiovascular System.* New York, Raven Press, 1979

West JB: *Respiratory Physiology—The Essentials.* 3d ed. Baltimore, Williams and Wilkins, 1985

Chapter 8

Integrated Cardiovascular Responses

The previous chapters have provided the building blocks necessary for understanding how the circulation works as a whole. This chapter is intended to encourage thought about how these building blocks fit together.

CARDIAC OUTPUT, VENOUS RETURN, AND CENTRAL BLOOD VOLUME

A key part of an integrated view of the cardiovascular system relates to understanding the relationship between cardiac output, venous return, and central blood volume. Consider the events that occur if the heart rate is suddenly increased by an artificial pacemaker (minimizing the changes in contractility that would accompany increased sympathetic neural activity). If the systemic circulation were a series of rigid pipes, the increased cardiac output would be instantly translated into increased venous return to the heart, and central blood volume would be unchanged. In reality, increased cardiac output raises pressure throughout the arterial circuit and causes an increase in arterial volume. This means that central blood volume is lowered slightly because some of the blood that would have returned to the chest is used to expand the arterial blood volume. This lowering of the central blood volume results in a diminished right atrial pressure and a diminished end diastolic volume. Stroke volume decreases and the increase in cardiac output caused by the elevated heart rate is not maintained.

Now consider what would happen if, just as the heart rate was increased, there was a slight venous constriction reducing the venous volume and just balancing the tendency for an increase in arterial volume caused by the higher cardiac output. In this case cardiac output would exactly equal venous return, and central blood volume would be maintained as would stroke volume; thus cardiac output would stay elevated. The point is that a transient difference in cardiac output and venous return results in a change in central blood volume. Central blood volume will affect cardiac output because of its influence on end diastolic volume.

THE CARDIOVASCULAR RESPONSE TO STANDING

A consideration of the cardiovascular response to standing (orthostasis) will provide an opportunity to consider the relationship between central blood volume, arterial and venous volume, and cardiac output in more depth. In general, standing causes intravascular pressures above the diaphragm to decrease and pressures below the diaphragm to increase (fig. 8-1). With quiet standing, right atrial pressure decreases from approximately 3 mmHg to 0 mmHg, and venous pressure in the feet increases by approximately 80 mmHg. Since these hydrostatic pressures are applied to both arteries and veins, they would have no effect on the flow between the aorta and the right atrium if the systemic circulation were made of rigid tubing. This is because pressure added to the venous side of the circulation (impeding flow) is exactly balanced by the same pressure added to the arterial side (enhancing flow). However, the systemic blood vessels (especially the veins) are not rigid, and they increase in volume with the increased internal pressure.

Consider what happens if an individual stands in water that is chest deep. Since water and blood have very similar densities, the hydrostatic pressure of the water on the outside of the body and the vessels will balance the hydrostatic pressure due to the column of blood on the inside of the vessels, and no increase in systemic vascular volume occurs. Cardiac output is therefore maintained.

What is the source of the blood that increases the extrathoracic blood volume? The major source is the central blood volume, which is reduced by approximately 400 mL when a 70 kg individual stands. This decrease in central blood volume would cause more than a 60% decrease in stroke volume and cardiac output if no compensatory mechanisms existed. With no reflex compensation, mean arterial pressure would drop by more than 60% and cerebral blood flow would fall, causing loss of consciousness. An adequate cardiovascular response to upright posture is absolutely essential to our life as a biped.

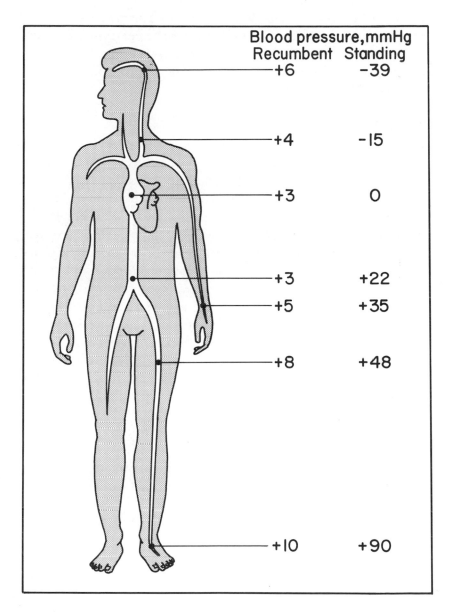

Blood pressure, mmHg	
Recumbent	Standing
+6	−39
+4	−15
+3	0
+3	+22
+5	+35
+8	+48
+10	+90

FIGURE 8-1.

Venous pressures in the recumbent and standing positions. In this individual, standing places a hydrostatic column of approximately 80 mmHg on the feet. Right atrial pressure is lowered because of the reduction in central blood volume. The negative pressures above the heart with standing do not actually occur because once intravascular pressure drops below atmospheric pressure, the veins collapse. These are the pressures that *would* exist if the veins remained open.

The cardiovascular adjustments to upright posture are (1) reflex increases in rate and force of contraction of the heart, and reflex arteriolar and venous constriction; (2) the muscle pump; (3) the respiratory pump; (4) myogenic constriction of arterioles; and (5) long-term adjustments in blood volume.

REFLEXES

The *reflex changes* in heart rate and force of contraction are initiated by the aortic arch and carotid sinus baroreceptors, and the volume receptors of the atria. When an individual stands, the increased venous pressure in the legs causes expansion of the leg venous volume (fig. 8-2). The blood for this increase in venous volume comes from the cardiac output that is trapped in the legs by the expanding veins. Thus for a few seconds venous return to the heart is lower than cardiac output. During this time, blood is withdrawn from the central blood volume. The decreased central blood volume results in decreased stroke volume and decreased cardiac output. The decreased mean arterial pressure and pulse pressure (due to decreased stroke volume) reduces baroreceptor nerve firing and leads to a reflex increase in sympathetic (and decrease in parasympathetic) neural activity from the medullary cardiovascular center to the heart. Heart rate generally increases approximately 10-20 beats per minute when an individual stands. The increased sympathetic neural activity to the ventricular myocardium shifts the ventricle to a new function curve, so despite the lowered right atrial pressure, stroke volume is decreased by only 40-50% of the recumbent value. These cardiac adjustments mean that cardiac output is reduced to 60-80% of the recumbent value. The increase in sympathetic activity also causes arteriolar constriction and increased total peripheral resistance. Mean arterial pressure may be increased to slightly above the recumbent value. A good question at this point would be to ask how increased sympathetic neural activity is maintained if the mean arterial pressure reaches a value near that of the recumbent value. In other words, why doesn't the baroreceptor nerve firing (and thus the sympathetic neural activity) return to recumbent levels if the mean arterial pressure returns to the recumbent value (or higher)? There are two reasons. First, although the mean arterial pressure returns to the same level or even higher, the pulse pressure remains reduced because the stroke volume is decreased 40-50%. As indicated in chapter 5, the firing rate of the baroreceptors depends on both the mean arterial pressure and the pulse pressure. The reduced pulse pressure means that the baroreceptor firing frequency remains lower even if the mean arterial pressure is slightly higher. Another reason is the continued low central blood volume, which means that the volume receptors of the atria fire less frequently and therefore cause increased sympathetic activity via the medullary cardiovascular center. Some investigators believe that it is decreased stretch of the atrial volume receptors that provides the primary afferent information for the reflex cardiovascular response to standing.

The arteriolar constriction caused by increased sympathetic neural activity does not reduce either coronary or brain blood flow. Thus the supply of oxygen and nutrients to these two vital organs is maintained.

MUSCLE AND RESPIRATORY PUMPS
Although standing would appear to be a perfect situation for increased venoconstriction (which could return some of the blood volume shifted to the legs to the central blood volume), reflex venoconstriction is a minor part of the response to orthostasis. Significant venoconstriction occurs only with more dramatic

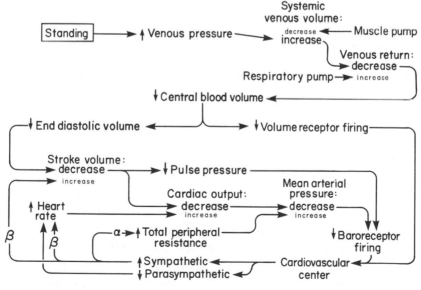

FIGURE 8-2.
Cardiovascular events associated with standing.

baroreceptor reflex activation, as with severe hemorrhage. However, two other mechanisms act to return blood from the legs to the central blood volume. The more important of these is the *muscle pump* (fig. 8-2 and fig. 8-3). If the leg muscles contract while an individual is standing, stroke volume increases to the recumbent value

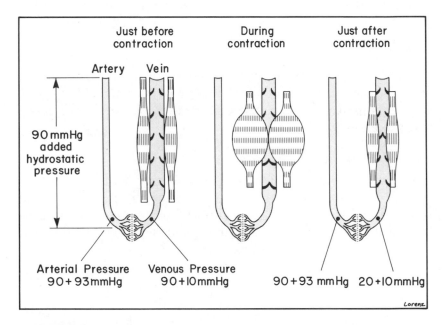

FIGURE 8-3.

The muscle pump. The muscle pump acts to increase venous return and to decrease venous volume. The valves (which are closed after contraction) break up the hydrostatic column of blood, thus lowering venous (and capillary) hydrostatic pressure.

very quickly. This occurs because of an increase in central blood volume that is caused by an increased venous return. The muscles expand as they shorten, which compresses nearby veins. Because of venous valves in the limbs, the blood in the compressed veins can flow only toward the heart. The combination of contracting muscle and venous valves provides a very effective muscle pump that transiently increases venous return as compared with cardiac output. Blood volume is shifted from the legs to the central blood volume, and end diastolic volume is increased. Even very mild exercise, such as walking, returns central blood volume and stroke volume to recumbent values.

The *respiratory pump* is another mechanism that acts to transiently enhance venous return and restore central blood volume (fig. 8-2 and fig. 8-4). Quiet standing for 5 or 10 minutes invariably

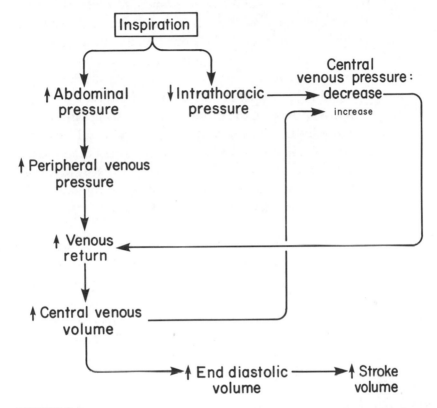

FIGURE 8-4.
The respiratory pump. Respiratory inspiration leads to an increase in venous return and stroke volume.

leads to sighing. This exaggerated respiratory movement lowers intrathoracic pressure more than usually occurs with inspiration. This fall in intrathoracic pressure increases the transmural pressure of the intrathoracic vessels and volume increases. The contraction of the diaphragm simultaneously raises intra-abdominal pressure, which compresses the abdominal veins. Since the venous valves prevent the backflow of blood into the legs, the raised intra-abdominal pressure forces blood toward the intrathoracic vessels (which are expanding due to the lowered intrathoracic pressure). This see-saw action of the respiratory pump tends to displace extrathoracic blood volume toward the chest and raise right atrial pressure and stroke volume.

CONSTRICTION OF ARTERIOLES

During continued quiet (minimum muscular movement) standing for 10 to 15 minutes, the baroreceptor reflex effects on the heart and the arterioles are not sufficient to prevent a lowered arterial pressure. Prolonged quiet standing causes an individual to faint as mean arterial pressure and cerebral blood flow fall. This vascular decompensation occurs because of effects of the elevated capillary hydrostatic pressure. The hydrostatic column of blood above capillaries of the legs and feet raises capillary filtration. Over a period of 30 minutes, a loss of 10% of the blood volume into the interstitial space can occur. This loss, coupled with the 400 mL displaced from the central blood volume because of redistribution of blood to the legs, causes central blood volume to fall so low that reflex sympathetic nerve activity cannot maintain cardiac output and mean arterial pressure; diminished cerebral blood flow and loss of consciousness result.[1]

Arteriolar constriction due to the increased reflex sympathetic neural activity tends to reduce capillary hydrostatic pressure. This alone does not bring capillary hydrostatic pressure back to normal because it does not affect the hydrostatic pressure exerted on the capillaries from the venous side. The most important factor counteracting the increased capillary hydrostatic pressure is the muscle pump. The alternate compression and filling of the veins as the muscle pump works means that the venous valves are closed a good deal of the time. When the valves are closed, the hydrostatic column of blood in leg veins at any point is only as high as the distance between the proximate valves. The combination of the muscle pump and arteriolar constriction reduces but does not prevent net filtration (fig. 8-5).

The myogenic response of arterioles to increased transmural pressure also acts against excess filtration. As discussed in chapter 7, raising transmural pressure stretches vascular smooth muscle and causes it to contract. This is especially true for the myocytes of precapillary arterioles. The elevated transmural pressure associated with standing causes a myogenic response and decreases the number of open capillaries. The fewer the number of open capillaries, the lower the filtration rate for a given capillary hydrostatic pressure imbalance (see chapter 6).

---

[1] You should now be able to describe the proximate cause of death by crucifixion.

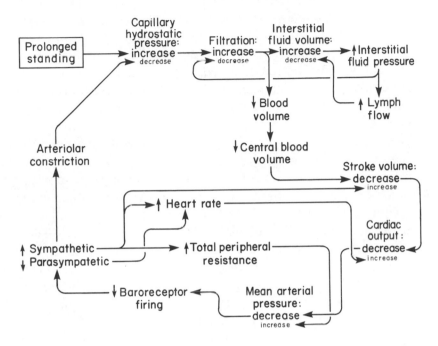

FIGURE 8-5.
Capillary and other cardiovascular events associated with prolonged standing.

In addition to the factors cited above, the safety factors against edema (described in chapter 6) play an important role in preventing excessive translocation of plasma volume into the interstitial space. The neural and myogenic responses, as well as the muscle and respiratory pumps, have been described. All play a significant role during the seconds and minutes following orthostasis.

LONG-TERM ADJUSTMENTS
In addition to these relatively short-term cardiovascular responses, there are equally important long-term adjustments. Patients confined to bed, or astronauts not subject to the force of gravity, exhibit a reduction in blood volume that begins during the first day or two and is quite dramatic after a week. Looking at it another way, maintaining an erect posture in the earth's gravitational field results in an increase in blood volume. This increase in blood volume is proportioned between the extrathoracic and intrathoracic vessels. The increased blood volume augments stroke volume during standing. In

the absence of this increment in blood volume, standing is extremely difficult if not impossible because of *orthostatic hypotension* (diminished blood pressure associated with standing). Orthostatic hypotension occurs, for example, in otherwise normal individuals who have been confined to bed, and in astronauts who have been out of the earth's gravitational field for some time. After a couple of days the blood volume returns to normal and so does the tolerance to the upright posture. There are many other causes of orthostatic hypotension, including hemorrhage and dysfunction of the autonomic nervous system.

The mechanisms responsible for increases in blood volume are initiated by the same afferent information that causes increased sympathetic nerve activity. The mechanisms responsible for the increase in blood volume are considered to be in the province of renal physiology. A detailed consideration of the renal mechanisms mentioned here can be found in texts on that subject. What follows is an overview of the factors responsible for maintenance of blood volume as they relate to the long-term control of blood pressure.

Plasma is a part of the extracellular compartment and is subject to the factors that regulate the size of that space. The osmotically important electrolytes of the extracellular fluid are the sodium ion and its partner, the chloride ion.[2] The control of the extracellular fluid volume is determined by the balance between the intake and excretion of sodium and water. Sodium excretion is much more closely regulated than sodium intake. The excretion of Na^+ can be controlled by altering (1) glomerular filtration rate, (2) plasma aldosterone concentration, and (3) a variety of "third factors" yet to be fully described (fig. 8-6). The important determinant of glomerular filtration is glomerular capillary pressure. This is dependent upon precapillary and postcapillary resistance and arterial pressure. When decreased mean arterial pressure and/or afferent arteriolar constriction results in lowered glomerular capillary pressure and less filtration of fluid into the nephron, sodium excretion tends to be decreased.

Aldosterone acts on the distal nephron to cause increased reabsorption of sodium and thereby decreases its excretion. Aldosterone release from the adrenal cortex is increased by (among other things) angiotensin II, the control of which was discussed in chapter 5.

---

[2]We will consider regulation of sodium ion balance alone, but an anion (usually chloride) always accompanies a sodium ion when it is gained or lost from the body.

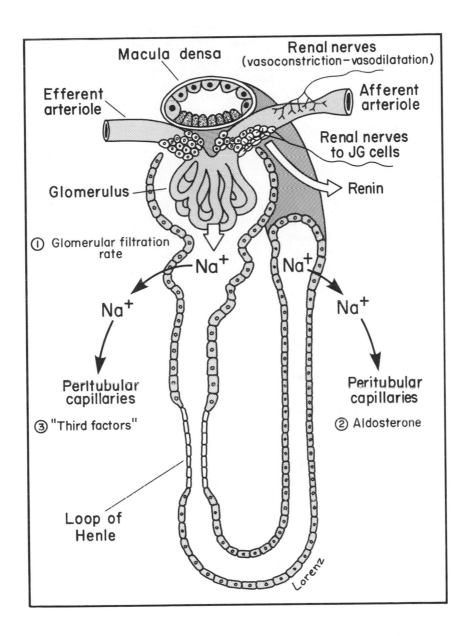

FIGURE 8-6.
Factors influencing renal sodium excretion.

Water intake is determined by thirst and the availability of water. Excretion of water is strongly influenced by vasopressin. Both thirst and vasopressin release are increased by increases in plasma osmolarity, which are sensed by certain areas of the hypothalamus. The same hypothalamic areas are also activated by decreased stretch receptor activity in the atria, as explained in chapter 5. Like increased osmolarity, decreased stretch receptor activity results in enhanced thirst and vasopressin release.

Consider how these physiological variables are altered by orthostasis and produce an increase in the extracellular fluid volume. Renal arteriolar vasoconstriction associated with the increased sympathetic activity produced by standing reduces glomerular filtration rate. The decrease in glomerular filtration rate results in a decrease in filtered sodium into the nephron and tends to decrease Na^+ excretion. The increased sympathetic nervous activity to the kidney also causes renin release, which increases circulating angiotensin II and in turn aldosterone release (see chapter 5). The decrease in central blood volume associated with standing reduces atrial stretch receptor activity, causing increased vasopressin to be released from the posterior pituitary. Thus both Na^+ and water are retained, and thirst is increased. The precise quantities of water and Na^+ can be adjusted to maintain the correct osmolarity of the plasma.

The distribution of extracellular fluid between plasma and interstitial compartments is determined by the balance of the hydrostatic and colloid osmotic forces across the capillary wall. Retention of Na^+ and water tends to dilute the plasma protein. The decrease in plasma colloid osmotic pressure would favor net filtration into the interstitial fluid. However, an increased synthesis of plasma protein by the liver occurs, so a fraction of the retained Na^+ and water contributes to an increase in plasma volume.

Finally, the increase in plasma volume in the absence of any change in total red cell volume decreases hematocrit, which can stimulate erythropoietin release and erythropoiesis. This may help red blood cell volume to keep pace with plasma volume.

Figure 8-7 summarizes the reverse process: the reduction in blood volume that occurs with prolonged recumbency, that is, bed rest. The decrease in blood volume that occurs in one week of bed rest is enough to make standing difficult for most individuals. With the decrease in blood volume, standing causes central blood volume to become too low to provide an adequate ventricular end dias-

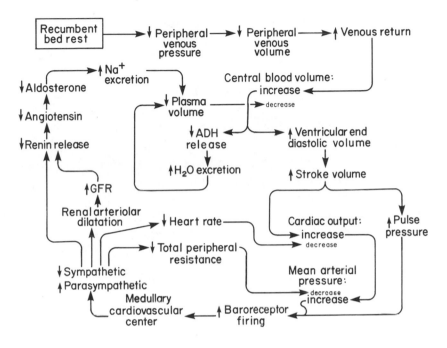

FIGURE 8-7.
Cardiovascular response to recumbent bed rest.

tolic volume. The reflex compensatory mechanisms are inadequate to maintain cardiac output and arterial pressure.

In situations resulting in the loss of extracellular fluid volume (such as sweating, hemorrhage, or loss of gastrointestinal secretions), restoration of normal plasma and blood volume depends upon these cardiovascular-renal mechanisms just described. Viewed in the context of the cardiovascular system, sweating and loss of gastrointestinal secretions are both losses of plasma ultrafiltrate, such as occurs with filtration from capillaries of the legs and feet with orthostasis (i.e., edema). Thus salt and water, but not plasma or red blood cells, must be replaced. Hemorrhage has many features in common with orthostasis. Hemorrhage reduces central blood volume. The effects on end diastolic volume, cardiac output, and mean arterial pressure follow from the decrease in central blood volume. The increase in arteriolar resistance resulting from the baroreceptor reflex coupled with the lowered mean arterial pressure decreases capillary hydrostatic pressure. This favors reabsorption of fluid from the interstitium and tends to increase plasma volume and reduce hematocrit. Replenishment of the lost blood involves the cardiovascular-renal events outlined above, as well as plasma protein and red blood cell synthesis.

EXERCISE

Exercise places the most severe physiological strain on the cardiovascular system. During heavy exercise, skeletal muscle blood flow may increase as much as 18 L/min from a resting flow of approximately 1 L/min. The increased blood flow to skeletal muscle is almost matched by an increase in cardiac output from 5.5 up to 22 L/min. The remainder of the blood flow is redistributed from the renal and splanchnic beds. The cardiovascular responses during exercise represent an orchestration of local metabolic effects in the heart and skeletal muscle, and centrally mediated effects on other organs.

The *anticipation* of exercise activates the defense response, with inhibition of parasympathetic and excitation of sympathetic pathways. Heart rate increases as does force of contraction. In some situations sympathetic cholinergic fibers to skeletal muscle arteries may be activated, leading to vasodilation before exercise begins. Circulating epinephrine may cause skeletal muscle vasodilation via β_2-adrenergic receptors. At least mild vasoconstriction of splanchnic and renal arterioles occurs. Skin blood flow is determined primarily by thermoregulatory reflexes and is little affected by the anticipation of exercise. The hypothalamic output partially overrides the medullary-cardiovascular center-mediated baroreceptor reflex, and mean arterial pressure increases by approximately 25%.

When rhythmic exercise begins, skeletal muscle arterioles dilate and blood flow increases in proportion to the increased oxygen consumption. The excellent correlation between cardiac output and whole body oxygen consumption is a reflection of the fact that skeletal muscle blood flow is so well matched to its oxygen consumption. The matching is due to the local metabolic vasodilator mechanisms such as K^+ and adenosine release, diminished tissue pO_2, and increased tissue osmolarity. The higher the metabolic activity of muscle, the more vasodilation. The cardiac output increases, holding the arterial pressure relatively constant and thereby maintaining the increased skeletal muscle blood flow. Capillaries open because of dilation of precapillary vessels. This means that diffusion distances are shortened and capillary surface area is increased, promoting better delivery of oxygen and substrate and better clearance of carbon dioxide and waste products.

Exercise automatically brings the muscle and respiratory pumps into play. Because exercise usually is performed in the upright position, central blood volume and stroke volume are increased by these pumps (fig. 8-8). Exercise in a recumbent position causes no change in stroke volume because central blood volume is already high. If the person is erect, the muscle pump begins with exercise and shifts blood from the legs to the chest, increasing central blood volume and stroke volume. Then, in both positions, stroke volume remains relatively constant and further increases in cardiac output are accomplished by increasing heart rate. It is important to remember that the increase in heart rate could not result in a higher cardiac output if contractility were not enhanced by the sympathetic nerves. The increased contractility also provides more rapid contraction and relaxation of the ventricles so that diastole is not shortened quite as much as would be expected by increased heart rate.

The increased cardiac activity causes release of vasodilator metabolites into the myocardium, and coronary blood flow rises in proportion to the increased cardiac oxygen consumption.

Exercise physiologists debate the question of just what limits maximum performance in tasks involving high oxygen consumption and high cardiac output, such as middle distance running and cycling. It has often been observed that top performance is correlated with maximum cardiac output. A good hypothesis is that the limit for increased cardiac output occurs because further increases in heart rate encroach upon diastolic filling too much and stroke volume begins to fall off. An upper limit for cardiac output means that a further increase in delivery of oxygen to muscle is not possible except by more complete extraction of oxygen from blood. This limit on the delivery of oxygen to muscle may well be the factor that determines maximum performance.

An inability to increase cardiac output limits the exercise capacity of many individuals with coronary artery disease. When cardiac performance is impaired by partial coronary artery occlusion, stroke volume often falls as heart rate increases, so that little increase in cardiac output is possible. This occurs because the absence of sufficient coronary blood flow, and therefore oxygen and

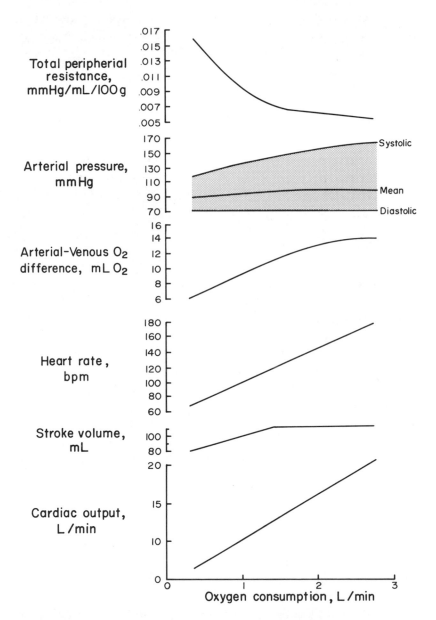

FIGURE 8-8.

Cardiovascular response to exercise during upright posture. Cardiac output increases as total peripheral resistance falls, with only minimal changes in mean arterial pressure. Stroke volume increases at low work rates and remains constant at higher rates. Heart rate increases linearly with increased work (bpm = beats per minute).

substrate delivery, prevents the increased contractility necessary to hold stroke volume constant. The performance of these individuals is limited, at least in part, by their inability to raise cardiac output.

When an individual exercises in a hot environment, thermoregulatory processes reduce the blood supply to skeletal muscle. Increasing core temperature causes increased skin blood flow, which diverts cardiac output away from skeletal muscle. Blood shifts from the chest to the skin, which exerts a negative effect on stroke volume. In addition, sweating reduces plasma and thus blood volume, and further reduces central blood volume and stroke volume. Thus maximum performance is limited by a hot environment, and patients with heart disease may find it difficult even to walk because of competition between thermoregulatory and metabolic demands on cardiac output.

Exercise involving the development of static, high forces, as occurs in lifting or shoveling snow, results in much greater increases in mean arterial pressure than does rhythmic exercise of the legs, such as in running, bicycling, or swimming. The increased mean arterial pressure in static, high-force work results from an elevated cardiac output in the face of a higher total peripheral resistance. The leg muscles involved in the exercise do not undergo metabolic vasodilation because the high-force development occludes intramuscular vessels. The increased sympathetic outflow associated with motor activities increases cardiac output and causes vasoconstriction of other vascular beds. Thus the increased sympathetic drive increases cardiac output with no accompanying decrease in total peripheral resistance; this means that arterial pressure rises a great deal. The adaptive value of this rise in mean arterial pressure may be that at least some blood flow is forced through the compressed blood vessels of the contracting skeletal muscle. The cost of this response is great, however. The increase in mean arterial pressure dramatically raises the oxygen consumption of the heart. This is far out of proportion to the exercise being done by the individual and reflects the much higher metabolic cost of pressure work by the heart. For this reason, static contractions of the large muscle masses may be especially dangerous for patients with heart disease.

Repeated bouts of exercise, such as running, bicycling, or swimming, result in a considerable improvement in cardiovascular performance. This training effect is reflected in a higher cardiac output.

The anatomic manifestation of this is enlargement of the ventricular chambers and increased wall thickness *(ventricular hypertrophy)*. An increased stroke volume results, and this means that a particular cardiac output can be achieved at a lower heart rate. The increased stroke volume raises the maximum cardiac output obtainable. The higher cardiac output of well-trained individuals does not produce an elevated arterial pressure, and this means that total peripheral resistance must decrease more than occurs in sedentary individuals. The increased vasodilation is due at least in part to an increased number of skeletal muscle vessels.

Two examples have been used—orthostasis and exercise—to show how the various elements of circulatory function are integrated to form a smoothly operating system with both short- and long-term controls. It is hoped that you have developed an overall view of the circulation something like this.[3] The variety of neural and hormonal cardiovascular control mechanisms are integrated to provide a relatively constant arterial pressure in most situations. Neural outputs are important in the moment-to-moment control of arterial pressure. The hormonal controls involving blood volume are important in the long-term control of arterial pressure. Arterial pressure is held constant by the correct adjustment of cardiac output and total peripheral resistance. The arteriolar tone of any organ or tissue is determined primarily by its function. In most cases local myogenic or metabolic mechanisms predominate in this control. (The skin is a major exception, where arteriolar tone is matched to function primarily by neural mechanisms. This relates to the special role of skin in holding body temperature constant.) Within wide limits cardiac output can be adjusted so that the blood flow needs of various organs can be met at a relatively constant arterial pressure.

Orthostasis gives us an example of the dominance of control mechanisms oriented toward control of mean arterial pressure because no special demands are placed on the cardiovascular system by an individual organ or tissue. Exercise gives us an example of change in the function of a tissue, skeletal muscle, which determines the performance of the cardiovascular system. The cardiovascular adjustments in most other circumstances are between these two extremes.

---

[3]This is in accordance with the dictum that a good teacher (1) tells the students what is going to be said, (2) says it, and finally (3) tells them what has been said.

Suggested Readings

Berne RM, Levy MN (eds.): *Cardiovascular Physiology.* 4th ed. St. Louis, The C. V. Mosby Company, 1981, pp 253-269

Guyton AC: *Textbook of Medical Physiology.* 6th ed. Philadelphia,W. B. Saunders Co., 1981, pp 332-355

Rowell LB: Circulation to skeletal muscle. In *Physiology and Biophysics.* 20th ed. Edited by TC Ruch and HD Patton. Philadelphia, W.B. Saunders Co., 1973, pp 200-214

Shepherd JT, Vanhoutte PM: *The Human Cardiovascular System.* New York, Raven Press, 1979, pp 156-179

Index

Index